ALZHEIMER & DEMENTIA

50 BRAIN FRIENDLY RECIPES

COOKBOOK

Meals that improve Memory and have the appropriate Nutritional value.

By CYNTHIA LEONARD

TABLE OF CONTENTS

DINNER OPTIONS: 67

SNACKS OPTIONS: 99

INTRODUCTION

Dementia and Alzheimer's disease are related disorders that mostly affect the elderly and impair memory and cognitive function. Here is a summary to aid in your understanding of them:

Definition of Dementia: Dementia is a word used to describe a set of symptoms related to a loss in cognitive function rather than a particular illness. Memory loss, difficulties with logic, communication and problem-solving are some of these symptoms.

Causes: A number of illnesses may lead to dementia, the most prevalent of which being Alzheimer's disease. Lewy body dementia, frontotemporal dementia, vascular dementia and other conditions are among the other reasons.

Symptoms: Depending on the underlying reason, dementia symptoms might vary, but they often include memory loss, confusion, disorientation, trouble speaking and interacting, poor judgement and behavioural or emotional changes.

Diagnosis: A healthcare provider will do a thorough assessment to determine the cause of a condition. This evaluation may include a patient's medical history, physical examination, cognitive tests, laboratory testing and imaging investigations.

Treatment: Depending on the underlying reason, dementia treatment varies. Many forms of dementia have no known cure, however treatments such as medication may help control symptoms and enhance quality of life.

Alzheimer's Disease Definition: Between 60 and 80 percent of dementia cases are caused by Alzheimer's disease. It is a slowly progressing neurodegenerative illness marked by the build-up of aberrant protein deposits (tau tangles and amyloid plaques) in the brain, which cause nerve cell death and a reduction in cognitive function.

Symptoms: Recalling names, conversations or recent events might be difficult to recall in the early stages of Alzheimer's disease. It can also be difficult to solve problems, focus or finish routine chores. The symptoms deteriorate with the illness and might include profound memory loss, disorientation, altered demeanour and trouble swallowing, speaking and moving around.

The biggest risk factor for Alzheimer's disease is advanced age, although other potential contributors include genetics, family history, lifestyle choices (such as nutrition, exercise and cardiovascular health) and environmental variables.

Diagnosis: In order to diagnose Alzheimer's disease, other possible causes of dementia must be ruled out using medical examination, cognitive tests and sometimes imaging scans or cerebrospinal fluid study.

Treatment: Cholinesterase inhibitors and memantine, among other drugs, may help some people with Alzheimer's disease temporarily manage their symptoms or halt the illness's course.

However, there is currently no known cure for the condition. Furthermore, patients' and carers' quality of life may be enhanced by support services, cognitive stimulation and lifestyle changes.

Comprehending Dementia and Alzheimer's disease is essential for prompt identification, efficient handling and assistance for those impacted by these illnesses and their family. We are still learning more about these illnesses and developing possible cures and preventative measures thanks to ongoing research.

BENEFITS OF NUTRITION FOR PATIENTS WITH ALZHEIMER'S AND DEMENTIA

For people with dementia and Alzheimer's disease, nutrition is important to their care and well-being. For those who have these problems, the following are some of the main advantages of a healthy diet:

Brain Health: The health and cognitive function of the brain have been related to certain nutrients. For instance, omega-3 fatty acids, which are present in fish, have been linked to a lower risk of cognitive decline and may benefit Alzheimer's patients with their memory and cognitive function.

Weight management: It's critical for general health, including mental health, to maintain a healthy weight. In those with Alzheimer's or dementia, proper diet may help avoid excessive weight loss or increase, which can improve overall quality of life and disease management.

Energy Levels: A healthy diet gives the body the energy it needs to perform at its best. Sufficient energy consumption may support people with Alzheimer's or dementia in continuing to be active and involved in everyday activities, which can improve their mood and general quality of life.

Nutrient Absorption: A lot of people with dementia or Alzheimer's disease may have trouble swallowing, eating or digesting food, which may make it harder for them to absorb nutrients from it.

Providing patients with easily chewed and swallowed nutrient-rich meals may help guarantee that they get the nutrients they need for optimum health.

Handling of Coexisting Diseases: Individuals suffering from dementia or Alzheimer's disease often also have other medical diseases such diabetes, high blood pressure, or cardiovascular disease. A well-balanced diet reduced in cholesterol, salt and saturated fats may help control these illnesses and lower the chance of problems.

Hydration: Staying properly hydrated is crucial for good health, particularly for those who may forget to drink enough water due to dementia or Alzheimer's disease. Regular fluid consumption is vital since dehydration may lead to various health concerns and a worsening of cognitive function.

Helping Carers: Healthy eating is beneficial to patients' carers as much as to the patients themselves. Serving wholesome meals to carers may lessen their stress and workload and enhance the general standard of care given to the person suffering from dementia or Alzheimer's.

Diet is essential to maintaining the health and wellbeing of those who have dementia and Alzheimer's disease. For patients and their carers alike, maintaining brain health, managing symptoms and enhancing general quality of life may all be facilitated by a well-balanced diet high in vital nutrients.

RECIPES

BREAKFAST OPTIONS:

Oatmeal topped with Berries and Chopped Nuts

Ingredients:

- ❖ Half a cup of rolled oats
- ❖ One cup of water or non-dairy milk
- ❖ A dash of salt
- ❖ 1/4 cup of mixed berries, including blueberries, raspberries and strawberries
- ❖ Two tablespoons of finely chopped nuts *(almonds, walnuts, pecans, etc.)*
- ❖ For sweetness, you may add *optional* honey or maple syrup.
- ❖ Cinnamon *(for flavour; optional)*

Instruction:

Heat a small pot over medium heat and add the milk or water.

Add a bit of salt and the rolled oats and stir.

Once the oats achieve the required consistency, reduce the heat to low and simmer them for around 5 minutes, stirring from time to time.

Cook the muesli for a few more minutes *if you'd like it thicker*.

After the muesli is cooked, take it off the heat and allow it to thicken for 1 minute.

After transferring the muesli to a bowl, sprinkle chopped nuts and mixed berries on top.

If desired, drizzle some honey or maple syrup over top for additional sweetness.

If preferred, add a sprinkle of cinnamon for extra flavour.

Serve your tasty muesli with chopped nuts and berries while it's still hot.

Feel free to alter this recipe by using other toppings, such chia seeds, shredded coconut or banana slices.

Greek Yoghurt Parfait with Honey and sliced Bananas

Ingredients:

- ❖ One cup of Greek yoghurt
- ❖ Two tablespoons honey or more according to taste
- ❖ One ripe banana, cut.
- ❖ 1/4 cup of granola *(more crunch if desired)*
- ❖ Fresh berries, **if desired**, as a garnish

Instruction:

Combine the Greek yoghurt and honey in a bowl and stir until completely blended. *If required*, add more honey after tasting to regulate the sweetness.

Place sliced bananas on top of the Greek yoghurt mixture in serving dishes or glasses.

Yoghurt may be layered at the bottom of the glasses, followed by a layer of sliced bananas and so on until the glasses are full.

Place a layer of granola, *if using*, over each layer of yoghurt and banana.

Once you get to the top of the glass, keep stacking and top with a layer of yoghurt.

If desired, garnish with fresh berries.

Serve right away or put in the fridge until you're ready to savour.

Scrambled Eggs with Spinach and Feta Cheese

Ingredients:

- ❖ 4 big eggs
- ❖ One cup of freshly chopped spinach leaves
- ❖ 1/4 cup of feta cheese, crumbled
- ❖ Salt and pepper.
- ❖ One tablespoon of olive oil or butter *(for cooking)*

Instruction:

Once the eggs are cracked into a mixing basin, thoroughly whisk them together. To taste, adjust the amount of salt and pepper.

In a nonstick skillet, preheat the butter or olive oil over medium heat.

Add the chopped spinach to the pan with the melted butter or heating oil. Cook, stirring periodically, until the spinach wilts, 1 to 2 minutes.

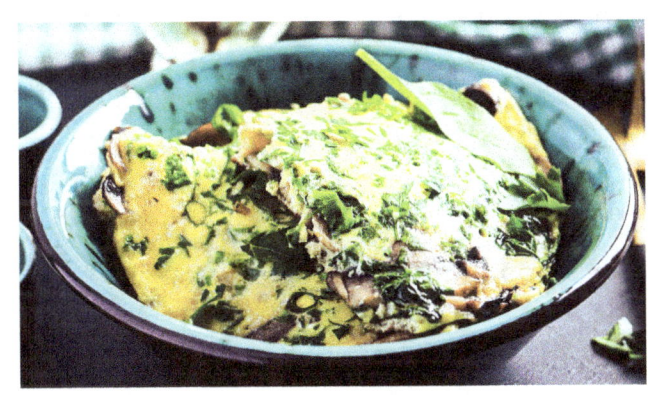

Transfer the whisked eggs and spinach to the skillet.

Allow them to cook for a few seconds - uncovered, until the edges begin to firm.

Using a spatula, gently stir the eggs and spinach combination, moving the cooked bits from the sides of the pan towards the centre.

Until the eggs are mostly set but still somewhat runny, keep heating and stirring.

Over the combination of eggs and spinach, scatter the crumbled feta cheese. To properly spread the cheese, give it a quick stir.

Cook for a further one to two minutes or until the cheese has melted slightly and the eggs are well cooked.

After taking the pan off of the burner, move the scrambled eggs with feta and spinach to serving dishes.

If preferred, add more salt, pepper or herbs to the garnish and serve hot.

Whole grain toast with Avocado spread and Smoked Salmon

Ingredients:

- ❖ Two pieces of whole grain bread
- ❖ One mature avocado
- ❖ One hundred grammes of smoked salmon
- ❖ Juice from lemons *(optional)*
- ❖ Salt and pepper.
- ❖ **Extra toppings at your discretion:** Cherry tomato slices, microgreens and slices of red onion

Instructions:

Get the Avocado Spread Ready:

Halve the avocado and scoop out the pit. Remove the meat and place it in a basin.

Use a fork to mash the avocado until it's smooth. To add some flavour and stop browning - pour in some lemon juice.

Add salt and pepper to taste while seasoning the mashed avocado. Tailor the seasoning to your own taste.

Toast the Bread

Toast the pieces of whole grain bread until they get crispy and golden brown.

Put the Toast Together:

Top each toasted piece of bread with a heaping tablespoon of mashed avocado.

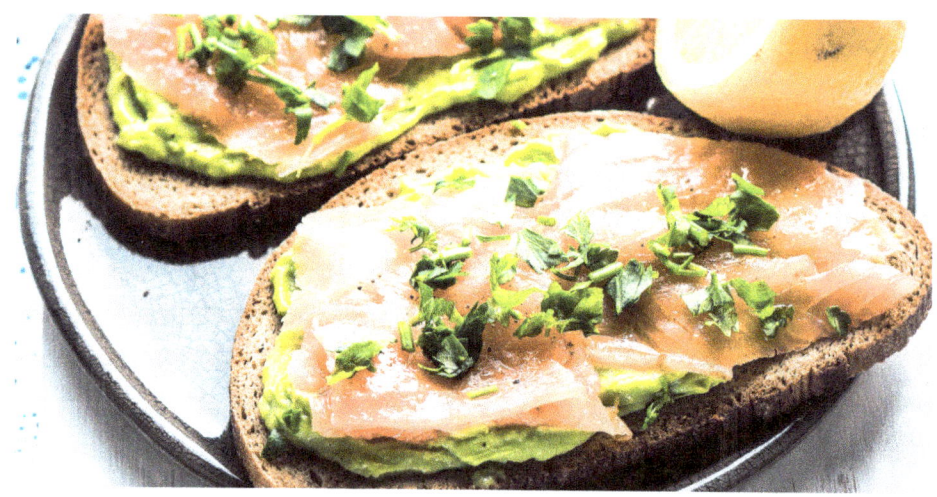

Arrange the smoked salmon pieces over the avocado mixture.

For added taste and texture, feel free to top with sliced cherry tomatoes, microgreens or red onion slices, **if preferred**.

Serve:

Your whole grain bread with avocado spread and smoked salmon is now prepared and ready to be consumed.

Serve it as a wholesome alternative for brunch, breakfast or a snack.

Smoothie made with Spinach, Berries, Banana and Almond milk

Ingredients:

- ❖ One cup of raw spinach
- ❖ Half a cup of mixed berries, including raspberries, blueberries, and strawberries
- ❖ 1 ripe banana, cut into slices and peeled
- ❖ 1 cup of unsweetened almond milk *(modify the quantity to get the right consistency)*
- ❖ **Not required:** *If preferred*, add 1 tablespoon of honey or maple syrup for sweetness.

❖ *Optional:* A half-cup of Greek yoghurt will boost the protein and creaminess.

Instruction:

Thoroughly wash the spinach leaves under running water, then pat dry.

Blend together the spinach leaves, almond milk, sliced banana and mixed berries in a blender.

For sweetness, add honey or maple syrup, for creaminess and protein - add Greek yoghurt.

To make sure all the ingredients are properly combined, scrape down the sides of the blender as necessary while blending on high speed until the mixture is smooth and creamy.

After tasting the smoothie, taste it and add additional honey, maple syrup or almond milk if necessary to modify the sweetness or consistency.

Once the smoothie reaches the right consistency, pour it into glasses and serve right away.

If you'd like, you can also top with more berries or chia seeds for more texture and nutrients.

Savour the nourishing and revitalising spinach berry banana smoothie.

Cottage Cheese with sliced Peaches and a sprinkle of Cinnamon

Ingredients:

- ❖ One-cup cottage cheese
- ❖ Slicing one juicy peach
- ❖ One-fourth teaspoon of ground cinnamon

Instruction:

Under running water, give the fruit a thorough cleaning. Slice it in half, then take out the pit.
Cut the peach into slender pieces.

Spoon the cottage cheese evenly over the surface of a serving dish or platter.

On top of the cottage cheese, arrange the sliced peaches.

Dredge the peaches and cottage cheese in ground cinnamon. Adapt the quantity to your own taste preferences.

Enjoy your tasty and nourishing cottage cheese right away with some sliced peaches and a dash of cinnamon.

It's easy to modify this recipe to your own flavour. For added taste and texture, you may also try adding a drizzle of honey or a handful of almonds.

Quinoa Porridge with diced Apples and Raisins

Ingredients:

- ❖ One cup of quinoa
- ❖ 2 cups of water

- ❖ One cup of your preferred milk *(dairy, almond or coconut milk)*
- ❖ 1 chopped apple
- ❖ one-fourth cup raisins
- ❖ Two teaspoons of honey or maple syrup *(optional)*
- ❖ 1/2 a teaspoon of cinnamon powder
- ❖ A dash of salt
- ❖ **Extra garnishes,** such finely chopped nuts or seeds *(optional)*

Instruction:

To get rid of any bitterness, rinse the quinoa with cold water through a fine-mesh strainer.

Rinse the quinoa and add water, milk, chopped apple,

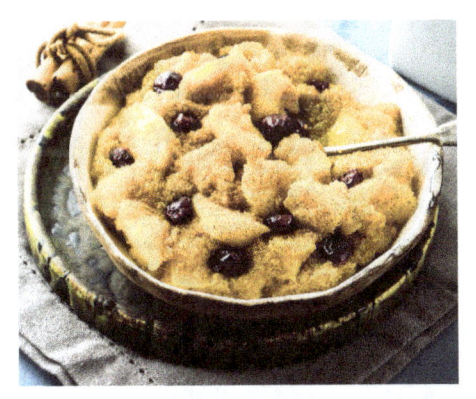

raisins, ground cinnamon, maple syrup *(or honey)* and a little amount of salt to a pot.

Heat the mixture on medium-high and bring it to a boil.

Once boiling, lower the heat to a simmer, cover the pot, and cook the quinoa for 15 to 20 minutes or until the porridge thickens to your preferred consistency.

To keep from sticking, stir from time to time.

When the porridge is cooked, take it from the fire and allow it to cool down a little bit before adding more thickening to it.

Top the heated quinoa porridge with more chopped apples, raisins, cinnamon and any other toppings you'd like, such chopped almonds or seeds.

Savour your healthy and tasty quinoa porridge topped with raisins and sliced apples.

You are welcome to modify the sweetness and spice amounts to suit your tastes. To add variation to the dish, you may also include additional fruits such as sliced bananas or berries.

Whole Grain Pancakes with Greek Yoghurt and fruit compote

Ingredients:
For the Pancake

- ❖ 1 cup of pancake mix
- ❖ One cup of flour made from whole wheat
- ❖ One tablespoon of sugar *(you may change this to suit your taste)*
- ❖ One tsp baking powder
- ❖ One-half tsp baking soda
- ❖ 1/4 tsp salt
- ❖ One cup of buttermilk *(or one cup of milk combined with one tablespoon of vinegar or lemon juice as an alternative)*
- ❖ 1 big egg
- ❖ 2 teaspoons of oil or melted butter
- ❖ One tsp vanilla essence

For the fruit compote:

- ❖ Two cups of mixed berries, including raspberries, blueberries and strawberries
- ❖ 1 to 2 teaspoons of sugar or to taste

- ❖ One tablespoon of lemon juice
- ❖ one-fourth cup water

For Serving:

- ❖ Greek yoghurt
- ❖ Extra fresh fruit *(optional)* for the topping
- ❖ *(Optional)* maple syrup

Instructions:

Get the compote fruit ready:

Put the mixed berries, sugar, lemon juice and water in a saucepan.

Over medium heat, bring the mixture to a simmer, stirring from time to time.

Simmer for 5 to 7 minutes or until the sauce has slightly thickened and the berries have softened then take off the heat and put aside.

Prepare Pancakes with healthful grains:

Mix the whole wheat flour, sugar, baking soda, baking powder and salt in a large mixing dish.

Beat the egg, buttermilk, melted oil or butter and vanilla essence in a separate dish.

Mix until just mixed, pour the wet components into the dry ingredients. Take care not to overmix; some lumps are OK.

Over medium heat, preheat a nonstick skillet or griddle. Apply a thin layer of butter or oil on the surface.

For each pancake, add about 1/4 cup of batter to the skillet. Cook for two to three minutes or until bubbles appear on the pancake's surface and its edges seem firm.

When heated through and golden brown, flip and cook for a further 1 to 2 minutes.

Grease the skillet as necessary and repeat with the remaining batter.

Put the Pancakes together:

Arrange a dish with a stack of pancakes.

Add a spoonful of Greek yoghurt on top. Over the Greek yoghurt, spoon the fruit compote.

Garnish with more fresh fruit, **if desired**.

If preferred, serve warm with maple syrup on the side.

Savour your nutritious and delectable whole grain pancakes paired with fruit compote and Greek yoghurt.

Vegetable Frittata with a side of Mixed Fruit

Ingredients for Vegetable Frittata:
- ❖ 6 big eggs
- ❖ 1/4 cup of cream or milk

- ❖ 1 cup of finely chopped mixed veggies - **including tomatoes, bell peppers, onions, spinach and mushrooms.**
- ❖ Half a cup of shredded cheese, either mozzarella or cheddar to taste.
- ❖ Salt and pepper.
- ❖ 2 tsp olive oil
- ❖ Fresh herbs for garnish, such as basil or parsley - *are optional*.

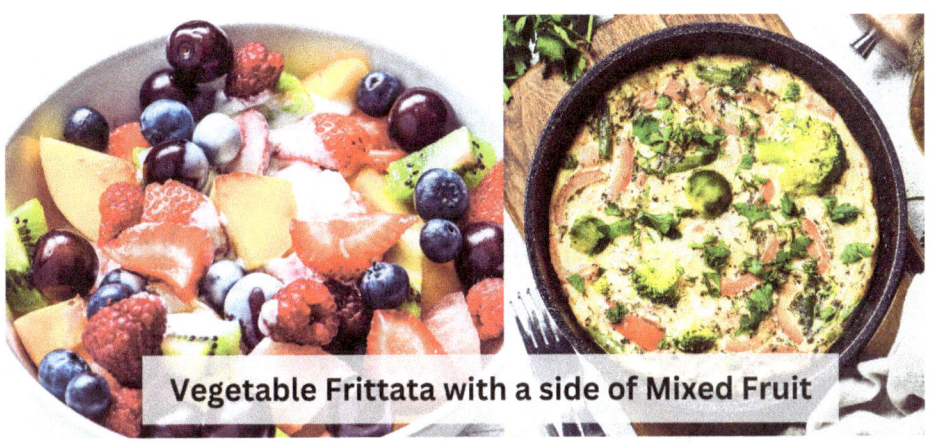

Vegetable Frittata with a side of Mixed Fruit

Instruction:

Turn the oven on to 375°F or 190°C.

Whisk the eggs, milk, salt and pepper in a mixing bowl until well blended.

In a large ovenproof skillet, heat the olive oil over medium heat.

When the mixed veggies are tender, add them to the pan and sauté for 5 to 7 minutes.

Over the veggies in the pan, pour the egg mixture. To spread the veggies uniformly, give them a little stir.

Cook the frittata over medium heat for 3 to 4 minutes or until the edges begin to firm.

Evenly distribute the shredded cheese on top of the frittata.

Place the pan in the oven that has been warmed and bake for 12 to 15 minutes or until the top of the frittata is gently browned.

After it's finished, take it out of the oven and give it some time to cool. **If desired**, garnish with fresh herbs.

Serve the frittata hot or room temperature after slicing it into wedges.

Fruit Salad with Mixed Ingredients:
- ❖ 2 cups of mixed fresh fruit *(mango, pineapple, kiwi, blueberries, strawberries and blueberries)*
- ❖ One tablespoon of maple syrup or honey *(optional)*
- ❖ Garnish with fresh mint leaves *(optional).*

Instruction:

Wash the fruits and prepare them as required. Cut up bigger fruits, such as mangos, kiwis and strawberries into bite-sized pieces.

Mix together all the prepped fruits in a mixing basin.

Drizzle the fruits with honey or maple syrup, **if preferred,** and toss lightly to coat.

If desired, garnish with fresh mint leaves.
Present the veggie frittata with a mixed fruit salad on the side.

Chia Seed Pudding with Mango and Shredded Coconut

Ingredients:

- ❖ One-fourth cup chia seeds
- ❖ One cup coconut milk or any other kind of milk you like
- ❖ One tablespoon of maple syrup or honey *(optional; taste and adjust)*
- ❖ One ripe mango, chopped
- ❖ Two teaspoons of coconut shreds
- ❖ Garnish with fresh mint leaves *(optional)*.

Instruction:

Chia seeds, coconut milk, **and if desired**, honey or maple syrup should all be combined in a mixing dish.

Mix well to blend. Verify that the chia seeds are not in any clusters.

To avoid clumping, whisk the mixture once more after letting it settle for approximately 5 minutes.

Refrigerate the bowl for a minimum of 2 hours or overnight, covered. As a result, the liquid may be absorbed by the chia seeds, which thicken into a pudding-like consistency.

Stir the chia pudding well to break up any clumps once it has set.

Chia pudding should be divided into serving dishes or jars for serving.

Add shredded coconut and chopped mango to the top of each dish. **If desired**, garnish with fresh mint leaves.

Enjoy your tasty and nutritious Chia Seed Pudding with Mango and Shredded Coconut, served chilled.

You can modify the sweetness or toppings to suit your tastes. For variety, feel free to add more fruits or nuts.

LUNCH OPTIONS:

Grilled Chicken Salad with mixed Greens, Tomatoes and Avocado

Ingredients:

- ❖ 2 skinless and boneless chicken breasts
- ❖ Salt and pepper.
- ❖ One tablespoon of olive oil
- ❖ 6 cups of mixed greens, including rocket, spinach and lettuce.
- ❖ Half a cup of cherry tomatoes
- ❖ 1/4 cup finely chopped red onion and one avocado
- ❖ **Optional:** Feta or Goat cheese crumbles for a garnish

For the Dressing:

- ❖ 3 teaspoons of olive oil
- ❖ Half a tsp balsamic vinegar
- ❖ One tsp Dijon mustard
- ❖ 1 minced garlic clove
- ❖ Salt and Pepper.

Instructions:

Set your grill's temperature to medium-high.

Add a little olive oil, salt and pepper to the chicken breasts' seasoning.

The chicken breasts should be cooked through and no longer pink in the centre after 6 to 8 minutes on each side of the grill.

Depending on the thickness of the chicken breasts, the cooking time might change. When finished, take them from the grill and give them some time to rest before slicing.

Make the salad dressing while the chicken is roasting. Mix the olive oil, balsamic vinegar, Dijon mustard, minced garlic, salt and pepper in a small bowl until well blended and set aside.

Mix the mixed greens, cherry tomatoes, avocado slices and thinly sliced red onion in a big salad dish.

After the chicken has had time to rest, thinly slice it.

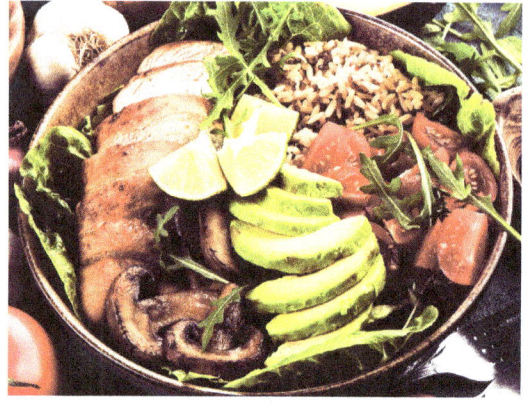

To the salad dish, add the cut chicken.

After one last whisk, pour the salad dressing over the greens. Gently toss to ensure that the dressing is distributed throughout.

If needed, adjust the seasoning by tasting it.

To add even more flavour to the salad, you may top it with crumbled goat cheese or feta.

Serve your tasty grilled chicken salad with mixed greens, tomatoes and avocado right away.

You can alter this salad to suit your preferences; for added crunch, toss in some toasted nuts or seeds.

Lentil Soup with Whole Grain Bread

Lentils Soup

Ingredients:

- ❖ 1 cup of dry lentils, any colour
- ❖ 1 onion, chopped finely
- ❖ 2 chopped carrots
- ❖ 2 chopped celery stalks
- ❖ two minced garlic cloves
- ❖ One can or fourteen ounces chopped tomatoes
- ❖ Four cups of broth made with vegetables
- ❖ One teaspoon of cumin powder
- ❖ One tsp finely ground coriander
- ❖ Salt and pepper.
- ❖ 2 tsp olive oil
- ❖ **For garnish**, use fresh parsley *(optional)*.

Instruction:

After giving the lentils a quick rinse in cold water, lay them out.

Heat the olive oil in a big saucepan over medium heat. Stir in the chopped celery, carrots and onion. Cook until the veggies are tender, approximately 5 minutes.

Add the ground coriander, cumin and minced garlic.

Once fragrant, stir and cook for an additional minute. Add the veggie broth and diced tomatoes then add the washed lentils and stir.

After bringing the soup to a boil, turn down the heat.

Cover and cook for 25 to 30 minutes until the lentils are soft.

Add salt and pepper to taste while preparing the soup. **If preferred**, top hot dish with fresh parsley.

Whole Grain Bread

Ingredients:

- ❖ 2 cups of flour made from whole wheat
- ❖ 1 cup of flour for all purposes

- ❖ 1 packet containing 2 1/4 teaspoons dry yeast that is active
- ❖ Warm water, 110°F/45°C - 1 1/4 cups
- ❖ 2 teaspoons of maple syrup or honey
- ❖ 2 tsp olive oil
- ❖ One tsp salt
- ❖ Extra olive oil *(optional)* for brushing
- ❖ Extra flour *(optional)* for dusting
- ❖ Oats or sesame seeds as a garnish *(optional)*

Instruction:

Mix the active dry yeast, honey *(or maple syrup)* and warm water in a large mixing basin. Give it a good 5 to 10 minutes to become foamy.

Stir the yeast mixture after adding the salt and olive oil.

Stirring constantly, gradually incorporate the whole wheat flour and all-purpose flour until a dough forms.

After transferring the dough to a floured surface, knead it for 8 to 10 minutes or until it becomes elastic and smooth.

If extra flour is needed to keep it from sticking, add it.

After the dough has doubled in size, put it in a lightly oiled basin, cover it with a fresh kitchen towel or plastic wrap and let it rise in a warm location for one to two hours.

Form the dough into a loaf by punching it down. Transfer the loaf to a baking sheet lined with paper.

For a further 30 to 45 minutes, lightly cover the loaf with a kitchen towel and let it rise.

Turn the oven on to 375°F or 190°C.
Not required: Drizzle the bread with olive oil, then top with oats or sesame seeds.

The bread should be baked for thirty to thirty-five minutes or until it is golden brown and hollow to the touch.

Before slicing, let the bread cool on a wire rack.

Savour a hearty bowl of lentil soup and some freshly made whole grain bread.

Tuna Salad stuffed in a Whole Wheat Pita with Cucumber slices

Ingredients:

- ❖ 1 can *(5 ounces)* drained tuna
- ❖ Mayonnaise - 2 tablespoons
- ❖ One spoonful of plain Greek yoghurt *(additional creaminess optional)*
- ❖ One tablespoon of lemon juice
- ❖ 1/4 cup celery, chopped finely
- ❖ 1/4 cup red onion, chopped finely
- ❖ Salt and pepper.
- ❖ Split 2 whole wheat pitas in half.
- ❖ Half a cucumber, cut thinly

Instruction:

The drained tuna, mayonnaise, Greek yoghurt *(if used)*, lemon juice, sliced celery and diced red onion should all be well mixed together in a medium-sized bowl. To taste, add salt and pepper for seasoning.

To make pockets, cut the whole wheat pitas in half.

Spoon a good portion of the tuna salad mixture into each opened pita pocket.

Place a couple cucumber slices over the tuna salad in each pita pocket.

Serve right away or pack each filled pita in foil or plastic wrap for a quick lunch.

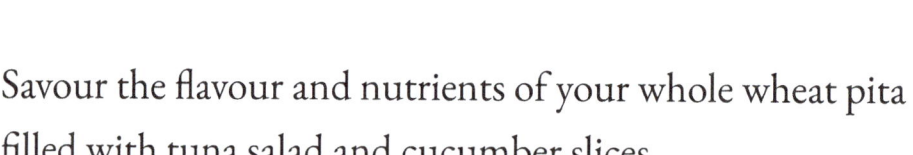

Savour the flavour and nutrients of your whole wheat pita filled with tuna salad and cucumber slices.

To add more crunch and flavour, feel free to alter the recipe by adding other ingredients like chopped tomatoes, shredded carrots or lettuce.

Turkey and Vegetable Wrap with Hummus

Ingredients:

- ❖ Four big whole wheat wraps or tortillas
- ❖ 1/2 cup hummus *(homemade or from the supermarket)*
- ❖ 8 pieces of deli turkey
- ❖ One cup of finely chopped lettuce
- ❖ Cut 1 medium Tomato
- ❖ half a cucumber, finely cut
- ❖ one-fourth of a red onion
- ❖ half a cup of shredded carrots
- ❖ Salt and pepper.
- ❖ Sliced avocado, sprouts or any other chosen vegetables *are optional*.

Instruction:

Arrange the tortillas in a neat line.

Leaving approximately an inch of space around the borders, evenly distribute about 2 tablespoons of hummus over each tortilla.

Arrange two turkey slices on each tortilla, overlapping them just a little bit if necessary.

Layer the turkey slices on top of the tortillas and equally divide the shredded lettuce, tomato, cucumber, red onion, shredded carrots and any other preferred vegetables.

To taste, add salt and pepper to the veggies.

Place sliced avocado over the veggies *if you're using one.*

To seal the contents within, securely roll the wraps, tucking in the sides as you roll.

If preferred, cut each wrapper in half diagonally or into more manageable bite-sized pieces.

Serve right away or for a handy grab-and-go alternative, carefully wrap each individual wrap in foil or plastic wrap.

Salmon fillet with Quinoa and Steamed Broccoli

Ingredients:

- ❖ 2 fillets of salmon
- ❖ One cup of quinoa
- ❖ 2 cups of chicken broth or water
- ❖ 2 cups of broccoli florets
- ❖ Two tsp olive oil
- ❖ two minced garlic cloves
- ❖ Salt and pepper.
- ❖ slices of lemon for serving

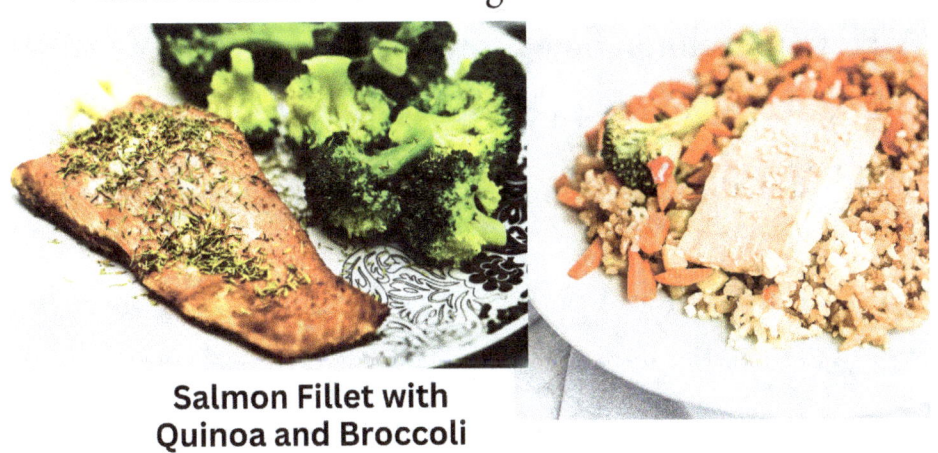

Salmon Fillet with Quinoa and Broccoli

Instruction:

First, prepare the quinoa. In order to get rid of any bitterness, rinse the quinoa in cold water.

Bring two cups of water or chicken broth to a boil in a medium saucepan. Turn down the heat to low and add the rinsed quinoa.

For approximately 15 to 20 minutes or until the quinoa is cooked and fluffy - cover and let simmer. When finished, take off the heat and use a fork to fluff.

As the quinoa cooks, get the salmon fillets ready.

Set oven temperature to 400°F, or 200°C.

Arrange the salmon fillets onto a parchment paper-lined baking sheet. Pour one tablespoon of olive oil and chopped garlic over each fillet.

To taste, add salt and pepper for seasoning.

Bake the salmon for 12 to 15 minutes or until it is cooked through and flake readily with a fork, in an oven that has been warmed.

Steam the broccoli while the salmon bakes.

To do this, set a steamer basket over boiling water, add the broccoli florets and cover with a lid. Steam the broccoli for 5 to 7 minutes or until it's soft but still has a vibrant green colour.

After everything is prepared, divide the baked salmon fillets, steamed broccoli and quinoa among your plates.

Before Serving, squeeze some lemon wedges over the salmon that is served alongside.

Savour your tasty and nourishing lunch.

Veggie Stir-fry with Tofu over Brown Rice

Ingredients:

- ❖ 1 block (14 oz) diced and drained firm tofu
- ❖ Two tsp soy sauce
- ❖ One tablespoon of sesame oil
- ❖ One tablespoon of cornflour
- ❖ 2 tsp of vegetable oil

- ❖ 2 minced garlic cloves
- ❖ 1 tablespoon finely chopped ginger
- ❖ One medium carrot, chopped into ribbons; one sliced red Bell pepper; one sliced yellow bell pepper
- ❖ 1 cup florets of broccoli
- ❖ Four cups of cooked brown rice
- ❖ One cup of trimmed snap peas
- ❖ One cup of sliced mushrooms
- ❖ Salt and pepper.
- ❖ **Garnishes optional:** Cilantro, green onions and sesame seeds
- ❖ 1/4 cup soy sauce is the sauce.
- ❖ Two tsp of hoisin sauce.
- ❖ One-tspn rice vinegar
- ❖ One spoonful of honey or maple syrup
- ❖ One teaspoon of Sriracha sauce or more according to taste
- ❖ One tsp of sesame oil
- ❖ Two tablespoons of water and one teaspoon of cornflour combined *(for thickening)*

Instruction:

Get the tofu ready: Cubed tofu, 2 teaspoons soy sauce, 1 tablespoon sesame oil and 1 tablespoon cornflour should all be combined in a bowl.

For uniform coating of the tofu, lightly toss.

To prepare the sauce, mix together all the ingredients in a small dish until well blended and then set aside.

To cook tofu, place a large pan or wok over medium-high heat with 1 tablespoon of vegetable oil. After adding the tofu cubes, heat for 5 to 7 minutes or until golden brown on both sides. Take out the tofu and put it aside in a skillet.

Stir-frying Vegetables: *If necessary*, add one more tablespoon of vegetable oil to the same skillet. Stir in the minced ginger and garlic for approximately 30 seconds or until fragrant.

Add the mushrooms, snap peas, broccoli, carrots and bell peppers after that.

Stir-fry the veggies for 5 to 7 minutes or until they are crisp-tender.

Put the tofu and veggies back in the skillet. Drizzle the tofu and veggies with the sauce. Once everything is well cooked and the sauce has somewhat thickened, give it one more good stir and simmer for a further 2 to 3 minutes.

Serve: Top cooked brown rice with stir-fried vegetables. If preferred, garnish with chopped cilantro, sliced green onions or sesame seeds.

Spinach and Strawberry Salad with Grilled Shrimp

Ingredients:
For the salad:

- ❖ 8 ounces of freshly washed and dried Spinach leaves
- ❖ 1 pint of freshly picked strawberries that have been cleaned, hulled and sliced.

- ❖ 1/4 cup of toasted almond slices
- ❖ 1/4 cup of optional crumbled feta cheese.

Regarding the Shrimps:

- ❖ One pound of big, peeled and deveined Shrimps/Prawns
- ❖ 2 tsp olive oil
- ❖ 2 minced garlic cloves
- ❖ one tsp lemon zest
- ❖ Salt and black pepper.

For the dressing:

- ❖ Balsamic vinegar, 1/4 cup
- ❖ 2 tsp honey
- ❖ One-fourth cup of extra virgin olive oil
- ❖ Salt and black pepper.

Instructions:

Set your grill's temperature to medium-high.

Mix the olive oil, lemon zest, minced garlic, salt and black pepper in a small bowl. When the prawns are added to the bowl, flip them around to ensure the marinade coats them evenly.

Give them ten to fifteen minutes to marinade.

In a separate bowl, mix together the balsamic vinegar, honey, extra virgin olive oil, salt and black pepper to make the dressing while the shrimps/prawns are marinating then set aside.

After marinating, thread the shrimps/prawns on skewers.

The shrimps/prawns should be pink and opaque after 2 to 3 minutes on each side of the grill. Take them off the grill and put them aside.

Toasted almonds, feta cheese crumbles *(if used),* cut strawberries and spinach leaves should all be combined in a big salad dish.

Pour the dressing over the salad and gently toss to ensure that all of the items are coated.

After dividing the salad among plates, sprinkle cooked shrimps/prawns over each portion.

Serve your delectable spinach and strawberry salad with grilled shrimps/prawns right away.

Whole Grain Pasta Primavera with Marinara Sauce

Ingredients:

- ❖ 8 ounces of full grain pasta, preferably multigrain or whole wheat.
- ❖ Two cups of homemade or store-bought marinara sauce
- ❖ 2 tsp olive oil
- ❖ 2 minced garlic cloves
- ❖ One small onion, chopped; one bell pepper; one zucchini; 1 cup cherry tomatoes, sliced;
- ❖ 1 cup florets of broccoli

- ❖ Salt and pepper.
- ❖ Grated Parmesan cheese *(for serving only, optional)*
- ❖ Chop some fresh basil leaves *(optional for garnish)*

Instruction:

Prepare the pasta:

Heat a big saucepan of salted water till it boils.

When the pasta is al dente, add the whole grain spaghetti and cook it as directed on the box.

After draining, leave the pasta aside.

Get the veggies ready:

Heat the olive oil in a big skillet over medium heat.
To the skillet, add the chopped onion and minced garlic.

Sauté the onion for 2 to 3 minutes or until it becomes transparent.

To the pan, add the broccoli florets, zucchini, cherry tomatoes and sliced bell pepper.

Simmer the veggies for 5 to 7 minutes or until they are soft but still crunchy.

To taste, add salt and pepper to the veggies.

Mix the Pasta with the vegetables:

Add the cooked pasta to the pan with the veggies once they're done.

Cover the spaghetti and veggies with the marinara sauce.

Mix everything together until the sauce coats the pasta and veggies equally.

Cook, stirring periodically, for a further 2 to 3 minutes or until everything is well heated.
Serve the Marinara Sauce-topped Whole Grain Pasta Primavera hot.

If preferred, garnish with chopped fresh basil leaves and grated Parmesan cheese.

Chicken and Vegetable Kebabs served with Couscous

Ingredients:

For the kebabs:

- ❖ 2 chicken breasts, skinned and boneless, chopped into pieces
- ❖ Cut one red bell pepper into pieces.
- ❖ One yellow bell pepper, chopped into pieces
- ❖ One red onion, sliced into pieces
- ❖ Rosy tomatoes
- ❖ Metal or wood skewers; *if wood, soak the skewers in water* for half an hour before using.

Regarding the Marinade:

- ❖ One-fourth cup olive oil
- ❖ 2 minced garlic cloves
- ❖ One tsp of paprika
- ❖ One teaspoon of cumin powder
- ❖ half a teaspoon of coriander powder
- ❖ Salt and pepper.
- ❖ One lemon's juice

For the Couscous:

- ❖ One cup of couscous
- ❖ 1/4 cup broth, either veggie or chicken
- ❖ One tablespoon of olive oil
- ❖ Add salt to taste.
- ❖ Freshly chopped Parsley *(garnish optional)*

Instruction:

To marinate the chicken, combine the olive oil, lemon juice, cumin, coriander, minced garlic, paprika and cumin in a bowl.

Toss to thoroughly coat the chicken pieces after adding them to the marinade. Allow the chicken to marinade in the fridge for a minimum of 30 minutes and a maximum of 2 hours, while keeping the bowl covered.

Prepare the veggies: Chop the veggies into bits while the chicken is marinating.

Put the Kebabs together: Set the temperature of your grill pan or grill to medium-high. Alternating between the marinated chicken, bell peppers, red onion and cherry tomatoes - thread the contents onto the skewers.

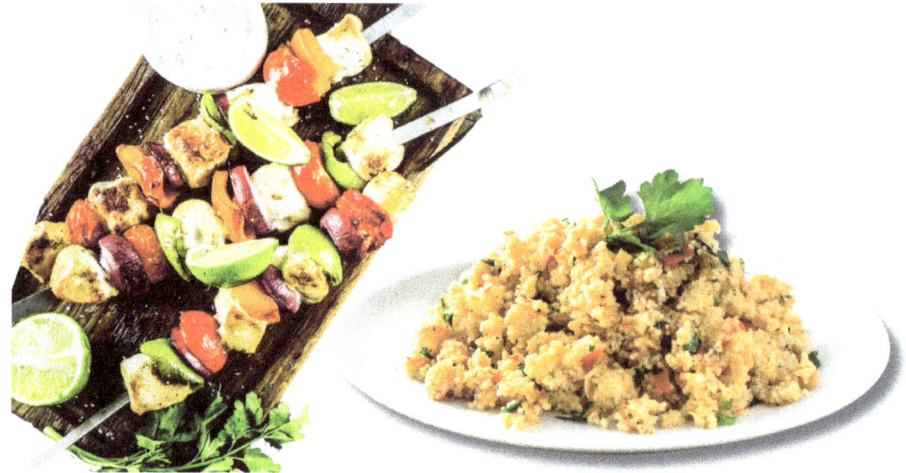

Grill the Kebabs: Arrange the assembled kebabs onto a grill pan or grill that has been preheated.

Cook the veggies for 5-7 minutes on each side or until they are soft and have a hint of char and the chicken is cooked through.

Prepare the Couscous: Follow the directions on the box to prepare the couscous while the kebabs are cooking. Usually, you will boil the broth, add the couscous, cover and remove the heat for five minutes.

Using a fork, fluff the couscous, then add a drizzle of olive oil and salt to taste.

Serve: Take the kebabs off the grill as soon as they are cooked through.

Serve the cooked couscous with the chicken and veggie kebabs. **If desired**, garnish with freshly chopped parsley.

Minestrone Soup with a side of Whole Grain Crackers

Ingredients for Minestrone Soup:

- ❖ Two tsp olive oil
- ❖ One chopped onion
- ❖ two chopped carrots
- ❖ Two chopped celery stalks and two minced garlic cloves
- ❖ One 14-oz can of chopped tomatoes
- ❖ One can (15 oz) of washed and drained kidney beans; six cups vegetable broth
- ❖ One can (15 oz) of washed and drained cannellini beans
- ❖ 1 cup of finely chopped green beans

- ❖ 1 cup of finely sliced zucchini
- ❖ 1 tsp of dried basil
- ❖ 1 tsp of dehydrated oregano
- ❖ Salt and pepper.
- ❖ One cup of elbow or ditalini-style tiny pasta

Complete Grain Crackers Ingredients:

- ❖ One cup of flour made from whole wheat
- ❖ One cup of flour for all purposes
- ❖ One tablespoon of honey or maple syrup
- ❖ One teaspoon of salt
- ❖ one-fourth cup olive oil
- ❖ half a cup of water
- ❖ Extra salt to provide a final garnish *(optional)*

Instructions:

For the Minestrone soup:

In a big saucepan, warm the olive oil over medium heat. Stir in the celery, carrots and onion. Simmer the veggies for 5 minutes or until they are tender.

Once fragrant, add the garlic and simmer for an additional minute.

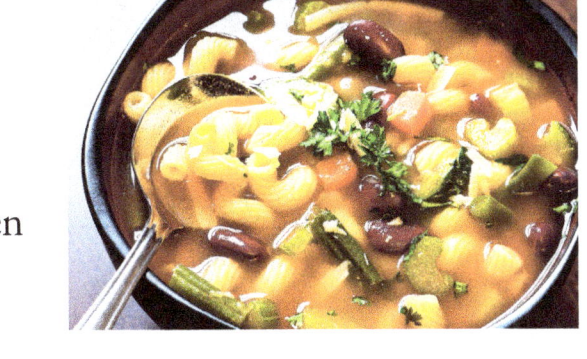

Add the zucchini, kidney beans, cannellini beans, green beans, chopped tomatoes, basil and oregano.
To taste, add salt and pepper for seasoning.

After bringing the soup to a boil, lower the heat and simmer it until all the veggies are soft - approximately 20 minutes.

As you wait, prepare the pasta as directed on the box. After cooking, drain and set aside.

After adding the prepared pasta, boil the soup for a further five minutes.

If necessary, taste and adjust the seasoning. Warm up the food.

About the Crackers Made Whole Grain:

Set oven temperature to 400°F or 200°C.

Mix the whole wheat flour, all-purpose flour and salt together in a mixing dish.

To the dry ingredients, add the water, olive oil and honey

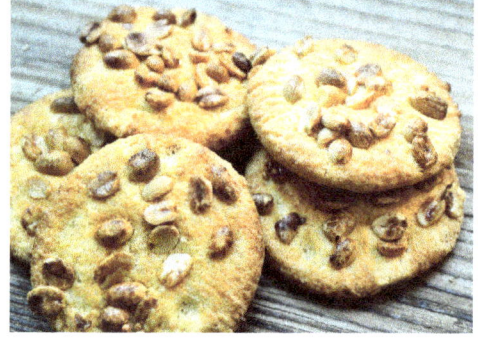

or maple syrup.

Stir to make a dough, then one spoonful at a time, add a little extra water to the dough if it's too dry.

The dough should be divided into two equal pieces. On a floured surface, thinly roll out each component.

To cut the dough into tiny squares or rectangles, use a pizza cutter or knife.

Arrange the crackers on a parchment paper-lined baking sheet. To stop the crackers from ballooning up, prick each one with a fork.

You may choose to add salt to the crackers' tops.

Bake for 10 to 12 minutes or until the crackers are crispy and golden brown, in a preheated oven.

Before serving the crackers with the minestrone soup, allow them to cool fully.

DINNER OPTIONS:

Baked Cod with roasted Sweet Potatoes and Asparagus

Ingredients:

❖ 4 fillets of cod
❖ Two big sweet potatoes, chopped and skinned
❖ One trimmed bunch of asparagus and two teaspoons of olive oil
❖ 2 minced garlic cloves

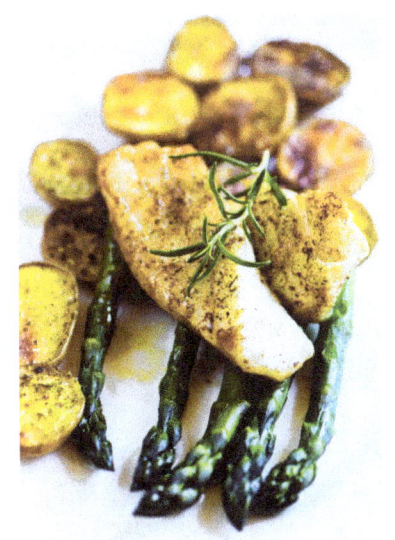

- ❖ One tsp of paprika
- ❖ One-half tsp dried thyme
- ❖ Salt and pepper.
- ❖ slices of lemon, for serving

Instruction:

Set oven temperature to 400°F or 200°C.

Arrange the sweet potatoes in diced form on a baking sheet.

Add a drizzle of olive oil and season with paprika, salt and pepper. For an even coat, toss - Make sure they are all in one layer.

Bake the sweet potatoes for approximately 20 minutes or until they are soft and beginning to turn brown, in a preheated oven.

Prepare the asparagus while the sweet potatoes are roasting. Transfer the chopped asparagus to a different baking sheet.

Add a drizzle of the leftover olive oil and finely chopped garlic. Add dried thyme, salt and pepper for seasoning and toss to evenly coat.

Roast the sweet potatoes and asparagus together for a further 10 to 12 minutes or until the asparagus is soft and beginning to crisp, after the sweet potatoes have been roasting for around 20 minutes.

Season the cod fillets with salt, pepper and paprika while the veggies are roasting.

When the veggies are nearly done, take the baking pans out of the oven and put the cod fillets on top of the vegetables that have been seasoned.

Place the baking pans back in the oven and continue baking for ten to twelve more minutes or until the cod is well cooked and flakes readily when tested with a fork.

Serve the roasted sweet potatoes and asparagus with the baked cod. **Before serving**, squeeze some fresh lemon juice over the top.

Beef Stir-fry with Bell peppers and Snap Peas served over Cauliflower Rice

Ingredients:

For the stir-fried beef:

- ❖ One pound (450 grammes) of thinly sliced beef steak
- ❖ One yellow bell pepper
- ❖ One red bell pepper
- ❖ One cup of snap peas
- ❖ 2 chopped garlic cloves and trimmings
- ❖ 1 tablespoon finely chopped ginger
- ❖ 2 tsp soy sauce
- ❖ One spoonful of sauce for oysters
- ❖ One tablespoon of sesame oil
- ❖ 2 tsp of vegetable oil
- ❖ Salt and pepper.
- ❖ **Garnish optional:** Sliced onions verde and sesame seeds

For the Cauliflower Rice:

- ❖ One head of cauliflower, chopped or blended into grains Similar to Rice
- ❖ One tablespoon of vegetable oil
- ❖ Salt and pepper.

Instruction:

Grate the cauliflower with a box grater or pulse it in a food processor until it resembles rice to make the cauliflower rice.

In a big skillet or wok, heat up one tablespoon of vegetable oil over medium-high heat. When aromatic, add the minced ginger and garlic and sauté for approximately one minute.

After adding the sliced beef to the pan, stir-fry it for three to four minutes or until it is browned and cooked through. After taking the steak out of the griddle, put it aside.

Add one more tablespoon of vegetable oil to the same skillet. Stir-fry the snap peas and bell pepper slices for two to three minutes or until they are crisp-tender.

Add the cooked meat and veggies back to the skillet. Stir in oyster sauce, sesame oil and soy sauce.

Toss to thoroughly mix in all the ingredients. Allow the flavours to combine by cooking for a further two to three minutes.

If necessary, add more salt and pepper to the seasoning after tasting.

In a separate pan, heat 1 tablespoon of vegetable oil over medium heat while the stir-fry is cooking.

When the cauliflower rice is soft but not mushy, add it and sauté it for five to six minutes, stirring often. To taste, add salt and pepper for seasoning.

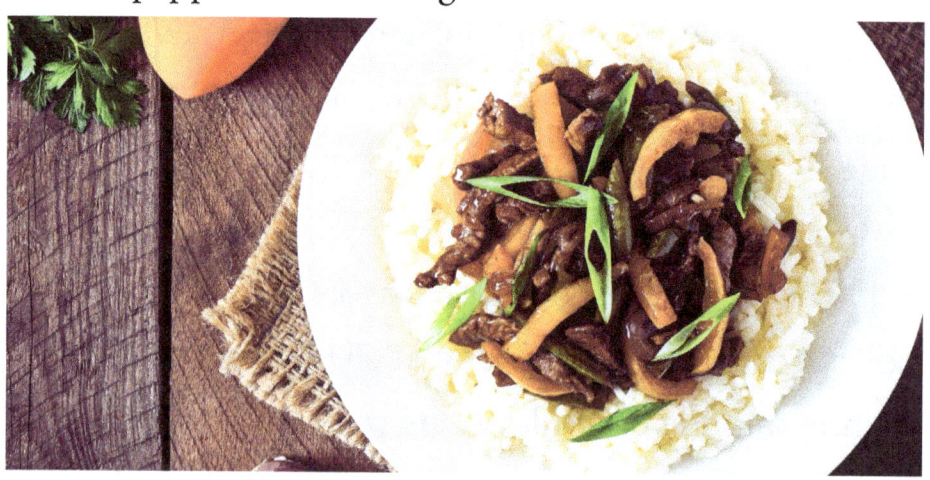

Over the cauliflower rice, serve the stir-fried meat. If preferred, garnish with sesame seeds and sliced green onions.

Savour the flavorful and nutritious stir-fried beef with bell peppers, snap peas and cauliflower rice.

Grilled Vegetable and Tofu Skewers with Wild Rice

Ingredients:
For the skewers:

- ❖ One block (14 ounces) of exceptionally firm tofu, compressed and diced.
- ❖ 2 Bell peppers, sliced into pieces
- ❖ Sliced one zucchini
- ❖ 1 yellow squash
- ❖ 1 red onion
- ❖ Chopped into bits 8 to 10 cherry tomatoes
- ❖ **To avoid burning**, immerse wooden skewers in water for at least half an hour.

For the Marinade:

- ❖ One-fourth cup soy sauce
- ❖ Two tsp olive oil
- ❖ 2 minced garlic cloves
- ❖ One spoonful of honey or maple syrup
- ❖ One teaspoon of cumin powder
- ❖ One tsp of smoky paprika
- ❖ Salt and pepper.

For the Wild rice:

- ❖ 1 cup of wild rice
- ❖ 2 cups water or vegetable broth
- ❖ Add salt to taste.
- ❖ **For garnish (if desired):** Lemon wedges, minced parsley or cilantro and fresh

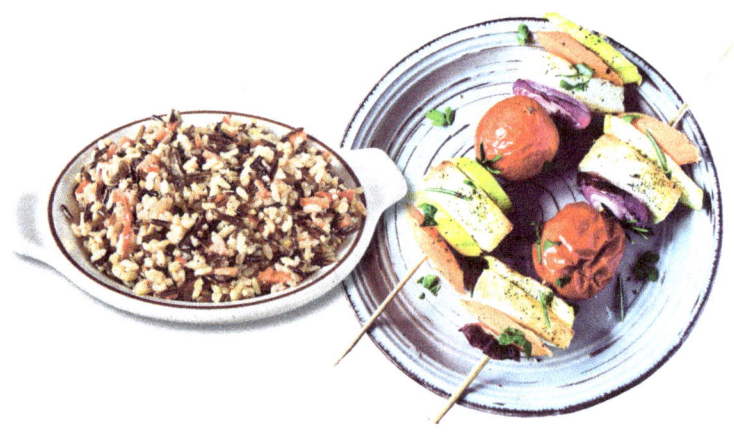

Instructions:

Mix soy sauce, olive oil, smoked paprika, ground cumin, honey, maple syrup and chopped garlic in a small bowl and season with salt and pepper.

Tofu cubes may be marinated by placing them in a plastic bag that can be sealed or in a shallow dish.

Make sure the tofu is evenly covered after adding the marinade. To enable the flavours to mingle, cover or seal the container and refrigerate for at least 30 minutes or up to 2 hours.

Rinse the wild rice in cold water to prepare it. Bring two cups of water or vegetable broth to a boil in a medium saucepan. Add a little teaspoon of salt and the washed wild rice.

Cover and simmer for 45 to 50 minutes till the rice is soft and has absorbed all of the liquid then turn down the heat to low.

When done, take it off the stove and cover it for five to ten minutes before fluffing with a fork.

Put the skewers together: Set your grill's temperature to medium-high. The marinated tofu cubes and prepped veggies are alternately threaded onto the wet wooden skewers with the tofu.

Place the constructed skewers onto the hot grill and cook them. Cook, stirring occasionally, for 10 to 12 minutes or until the tofu is well cooked and the veggies are soft and gently browned.

Serve: Arrange the cooked wild rice over a bed of grilled veggie and tofu skewers. Serve with lemon wedges on the side for squeezing over the skewers and garnish with chopped cilantro or parsley, **if preferred**.

Turkey Chili with Mixed Beans and a side of Cornbread

Ingredients for Turkey Chilli:

- ❖ One tablespoon of olive oil
- ❖ One pound of turkey, ground
- ❖ 1 sliced onion
- ❖ 3 minced garlic cloves
- ❖ One sliced red bell pepper
- ❖ One chopped green bell pepper
- ❖ Diced tomatoes from one can (14.5 ounces)
- ❖ One fifteen-ounce can of mixed beans *(pinto, black and kidney beans)*, washed and drained
- ❖ Two cups broth, either veggie or chicken
- ❖ 2 tsp of chilli powder
- ❖ One teaspoon of cumin powder
- ❖ One tsp of paprika
- ❖ Salt and pepper.
- ❖ Extra toppings at your discretion: sour cream, sliced avocado, chopped cilantro and grated cheese

Cornmeal Components:

- ❖ One cup of cornmeal
- ❖ One cup of flour for all purposes
- ❖ 1/4 cup of sugar, granulated
- ❖ One-third tsp baking powder
- ❖ Half a teaspoon of salt
- ❖ 1 cup of milk
- ❖ 1/4 cup melted unsalted butter
- ❖ One egg

Instructions:

For the Turkey Chilli:

In a big saucepan or Dutch oven, warm up the olive oil over medium heat.

Add the ground turkey and cook, breaking it up with a spoon as it cooks for approximately 5 to 7 minutes or until browned.

Add diced bell peppers, chopped onion and garlic to the saucepan. Simmer the veggies for 5 minutes or until they are tender.

Add the chopped tomatoes, mixed beans, broth *(either chicken or vegetable)*, paprika, ground cumin, chilli powder and salt and pepper.

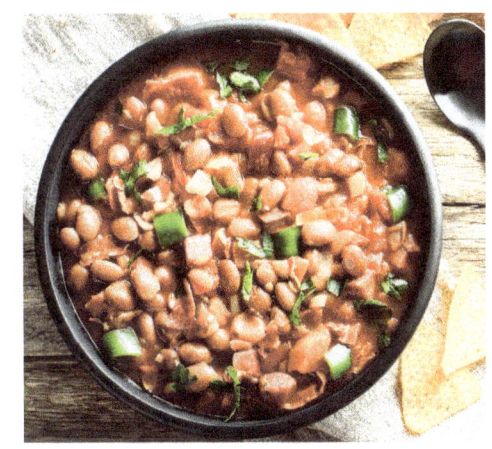

After bringing the chilli to a simmer, turn down the heat and continue to simmer - uncovered, stirring periodically for 20 to 25 minutes or until the chilli has thickened.

If needed, adjust the seasoning by tasting it. You may add some spicy sauce or a dash of cayenne pepper if you want your chilli hotter.

Serve the hot turkey chilli with your preferred toppings on top.

Regarding Cornbread:
Set oven temperature to 400°F or 200°C.
A 9 × 9-inch baking pan may be lined with parchment paper or greased.

Mix the cornmeal, flour, sugar, baking powder and salt in a large mixing dish.

Beat the egg, melted butter and milk together well in a separate basin.

Mix until well combined then pour the wet components into the dry ingredients. Take care not to overmix; a little lumpiness in the batter is OK.

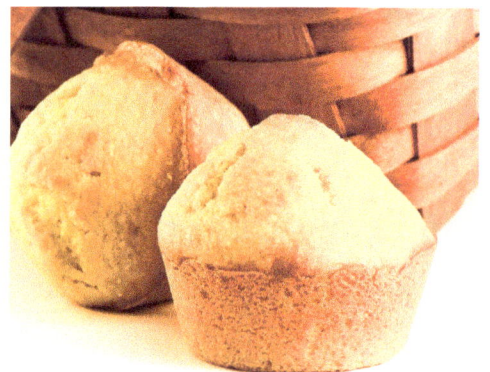

Using a spatula, level the top of the batter after it has been poured into the baking pan.

When a toothpick put into the centre of the cornbread comes out clean, it has been baked for 20 to 25 minutes or until it is golden brown.

Before cutting into slices and serving with the turkey chilli, let the cornbread cool somewhat.

Baked Chicken Breast with Quinoa and Roasted Brussels Sprouts

Ingredients:

- ❖ Two skinless and boneless chicken breasts
- ❖ One cup of washed quinoa
- ❖ Double-cupped Brussels sprouts, cut in half
- ❖ Two tsp olive oil
- ❖ 2 minced garlic cloves
- ❖ A single tsp of dried thyme
- ❖ One tsp of dehydrated rosemary
- ❖ Salt and pepper.
- ❖ slices of lemon *(optional for serving)*

Instruction:

Set oven temperature to 400°F, or 200°C.

Salt, pepper and half of the minced garlic should be used to season the chicken breasts.

The quinoa, Brussels sprouts, remaining minced garlic, dried thyme, dried rosemary, olive oil, salt and pepper should all be combined in a large baking dish.

Mix everything until well incorporated.

Top the Quinoa and Brussels sprouts mixture in the baking dish with the seasoned chicken breasts.

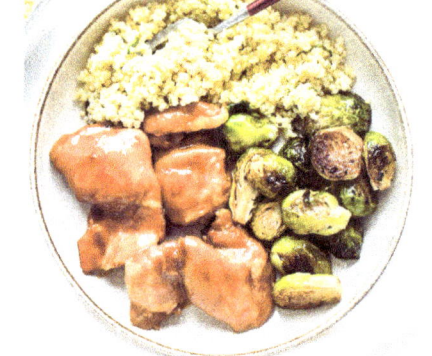

After covering the baking dish with aluminium foil, bake it in the preheated oven for 25 to 30 minutes or until the quinoa is soft and the chicken is well cooked.

For the last 5 minutes of baking, take off the foil to let the chicken gently brown.

Take the dish out of the oven as soon as the chicken is cooked through and the Brussels sprouts and quinoa are soft.

Serve the quinoa and roasted Brussels sprouts with the cooked chicken breasts.

If preferred, drizzle the chicken and veggies with freshly squeezed lemon juice just before serving.

Eggplant Parmesan served with Whole Wheat Spaghetti

Ingredients:
For the Parmesan Eggplant:

- One big aubergine, cut into rounds of half an inch
- Salt
- One cup of flour for all purposes
- 2 beaten eggs
- One cup of breadcrumbs *(for a healthy alternative, use whole wheat breadcrumbs)*
- Grated Parmesan cheese - 1 cup
- Two cups of marinara sauce
- Two cups of mozzarella cheese, shredded
- Olive oil for frying

For the Whole Wheat Pasta:

- ❖ Whole wheat spaghetti, 8 ounces
- ❖ For Pasta - Water and Salt.
- ❖ Extra virgin olive oil
- ❖ Chop some fresh basil leaves *(optional)*

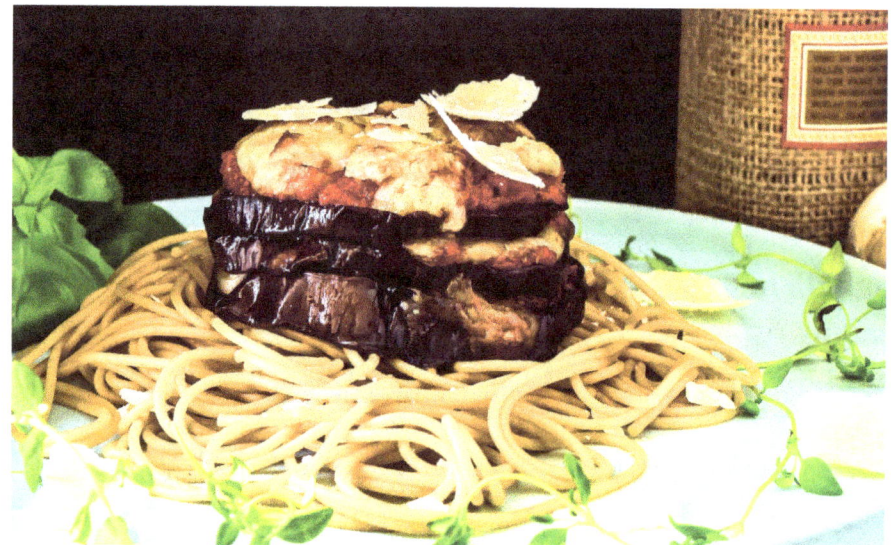

Instructions:

Turn the oven on to 375°F, or 190°C.

Arrange the slices of eggplant onto a baking sheet and lightly dust them with salt. Give them ten to fifteen minutes to sit.

This aids in removing the eggplant's extra moisture and bitterness.

Using paper towels, blot the eggplant slices dry once the allotted time has passed.

Arrange three shallow dishes: one containing flour, another containing beaten eggs and a 3rd with a blend of breadcrumbs and grated Parmesan cheese for breading the eggplant.

In a large skillet, heat a thin coating of olive oil over medium heat.

Each eggplant slice should first be coated uniformly with the breadcrumb-Parmesan mixture before being dipped in the beaten eggs and flour.

Cook the breaded eggplant slices in the pan until they are crispy and golden brown, approximately 2 to 3 minutes each side - *Fry them in batches if necessary*.

To drain any extra oil, move the fried eggplant slices to a platter covered with paper towels.

Line the bottom of a baking dish with a thin layer of marinara sauce.

Arrange a layer of sauce over the fried eggplant pieces. Continue layering and then pour marinara sauce over top.

Over the marinara sauce, scatter the shredded mozzarella cheese.

Bake the eggplant parmesan for 25 to 30 minutes in a preheated oven or until the cheese is bubbling and melted.

As the eggplant parmesan bakes, prepare the whole wheat spaghetti in a saucepan of boiling salted water, following the directions on the box.

To avoid sticking, drain the cooked spaghetti and mix it with a little olive oil.

Serve the whole wheat spaghetti with the heated eggplant parmesan. **If desired**, garnish with finely chopped fresh basil leaves.

Grilled Shrimp and Vegetable kabobs with Quinoa Pilaf

Ingredients:
For the Vegetable and Shrimp Kabobs:

- ❖ One pound of big, peeled and deveined prawns
- ❖ Two bell peppers, chopped into bits (*for visual interest, use various colours*)
- ❖ One red onion, sliced into pieces
- ❖ One sliced courgette
- ❖ One yellow squash, chopped
- ❖ 8 to 10 Cherry tomatoes
- ❖ Metal or wood skewers

For the Marinade:

- ❖ one-fourth cup olive oil
- ❖ 2 minced garlic cloves

- ❖ 2 tsp lemon juice
- ❖ One tsp of dehydrated oregano
- ❖ One tsp of paprika
- ❖ Salt and pepper.

For the Pilaf with Quinoa:

- ❖ One cup of washed quinoa
- ❖ 2 cups water or vegetable broth
- ❖ 1 tablespoon of olive oil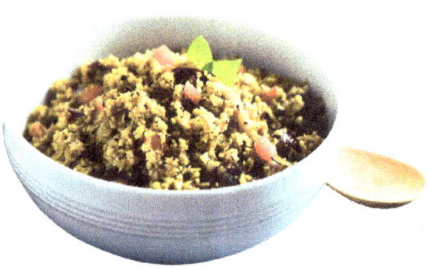
- ❖ 1 little onion, diced finely
- ❖ 2 minced garlic cloves
- ❖ half a cup of carrots, chopped
- ❖ half a cup of bell pepper, chopped
- ❖ half a cup of frozen peas
- ❖ Salt and pepper.
- ❖ Two teaspoons of finely chopped fresh parsley *(for garnish only)*

Instructions:

Combine all of the marinade's ingredients in a small bowl.

Pour the marinade over the prawns in a shallow dish and toss to coat evenly. Give it a cover and chill for a minimum of half an hour.

Make the quinoa pilaf while the shrimp are marinating.

Heat the olive oil in a medium-sized saucepan over medium heat. Add the chopped onion and simmer for 3–4 minutes or until transparent.

Cook for a further minute after adding the minced garlic.

Add the chopped bell pepper and carrots, stir and simmer for 2 to 3 minutes or until the carrots start to soften. Rinse the quinoa and add it to the pan. Toast it for 2 to 3 minutes, stirring often.

Add the water or veggie broth and heat until it boils. Once the quinoa is cooked and the liquid has been absorbed, reduce the heat to low, cover and simmer for 15 to 20 minutes. Using a fork, fluff.

As the quinoa cooks, have the skewers ready. Set your grill's temperature to medium-high.

Alternately thread bell peppers, onions, zucchini, squash and cherry tomatoes along with the marinated shrimp on skewers.

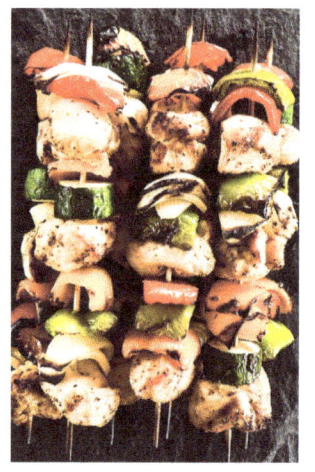

The shrimp should be pink and opaque and the veggies should be soft and gently browned after grilling the kabobs for 2 to 3 minutes on each side.

Serve the quinoa pilaf with the grilled shrimp and veggie kabobs on top - *if like*, top with chopped parsley.

Stuffed Bell Peppers with Ground Turkey and Brown Rice

Ingredients:

- ❖ 4 big bell peppers, any hue
- ❖ 1 pound of turkey, ground
- ❖ 1 cup of brown rice, cooked
- ❖ 1 little onion, diced finely
- ❖ 2 minced garlic cloves
- ❖ One can (14.5 oz) drained and chopped tomatoes
- ❖ One cup of finely shredded mozzarella cheese
- ❖ One tsp of dehydrated oregano
- ❖ One tsp of dried basil
- ❖ Salt and pepper.
- ❖ Olive oil

Instruction:

Turn the oven on to 375°F, or 190°C.

Slice off the bell peppers' tops, then take out the seeds and membranes. After rinsing them with cold water, put them aside.

One tablespoon of olive oil should be heated over medium heat in a skillet. Cook the minced garlic and diced onion for two to three minutes or until the ingredients are tender.

Using a spatula, add the ground turkey to the pan and

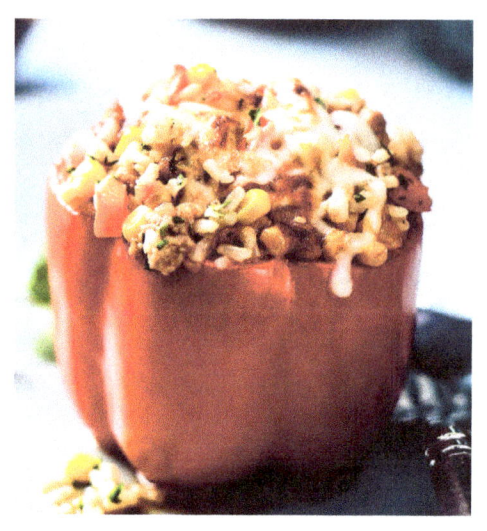 cook it for 5 to 7 minutes or until it is browned and well cooked.

Add the diced tomatoes, cooked brown rice, salt, pepper, dried oregano and dried basil and stir. To give the flavours time to mingle, cook for a further 2 to 3 minutes.

Bell peppers should be arranged vertically in a baking dish.

Fill each pepper completely by equally spooning in the turkey and rice mixture.

Over the tops of the filled peppers, scatter shredded mozzarella cheese.

Bake the baking dish in the preheated oven for 25 to 30 minutes, or until the peppers are soft, covered with aluminium foil.

After taking off the foil, bake for a further 5 to 10 minutes or until the cheese is bubbling and melted.

Before serving, carefully take the stuffed peppers out of the oven and allow them to cool for a few minutes.

If preferred, top the hot filled bell peppers with finely chopped fresh herbs like basil or parsley.

Baked Salmon with steamed Green Beans and Quinoa

Ingredients:
For the salmon:

- ❖ 4 six-ounce salmon fillets each
- ❖ Two tsp olive oil
- ❖ 2 minced garlic cloves
- ❖ 1 tsp lemon zest
- ❖ One tablespoon of lemon juice
- ❖ Salt and pepper.
- ❖ Chopped fresh herbs *(parsley, dill or thyme)*

Regarding the Green beans:
- ❖ One pound of cleaned Green beans
- ❖ Salt to taste.
- ❖ slices of lemon to serve *(optional)*

For the Quinoa:
- ❖ One cup of quinoa
- ❖ 2 cups of veggie broth or water
- ❖ Salt to taste.

Instructions:

Set oven temperature to 400°F or 200°C.

Rinse the quinoa with a fine-mesh strainer under cold water. Add the quinoa to water or broth - and a little amount of salt in a medium pot.

Over medium-high heat, bring to a boil. After that, lower the heat to a simmer, cover and cook for about 15 minutes or until the quinoa is tender and the liquid has been absorbed.

Take it off the heat and leave it covered for five minutes. Use a fork to fluff before serving.

As the quinoa cooks, get the fish ready.

Combine the olive oil, minced garlic, lemon zest, lemon juice, salt and pepper in a small bowl.

Arrange the salmon fillets on a baking sheet that has been gently oiled or covered with parchment paper. Make sure the salmon fillets are uniformly coated by brushing them with the olive oil mixture.

For 12 to 15 minutes or until the salmon is cooked through and flakes readily with a fork - bake it in the preheated oven.

Depending on the thickness of the fillets, cooking times might vary.

After trimming, put the green beans in a steamer basket over a boiling pot of water. For 5 to 7 minutes or when the green beans are soft but still crunchy, cover and steam the beans.

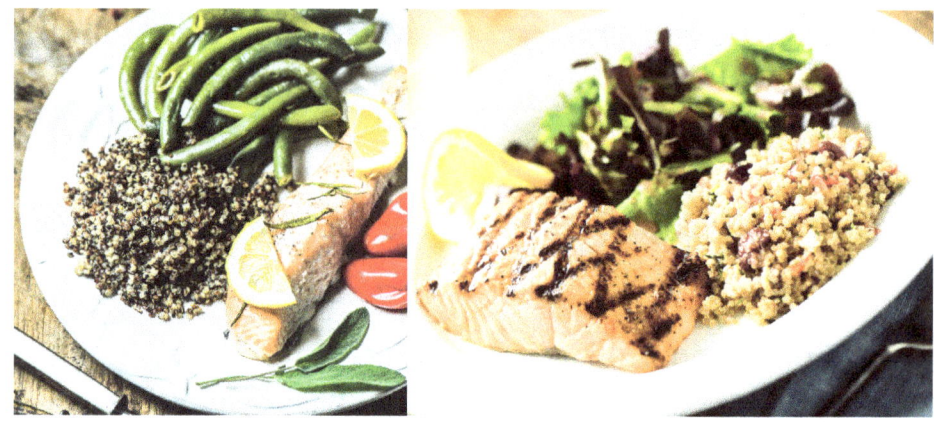

After everything is cooked, transfer the green beans, salmon and quinoa to individual serving dishes.

If preferred, serve with lemon wedges on the side and garnish with fresh herbs and serve.

You are welcome to modify the ingredients and spices to suit your tastes.

Vegetable Curry with Chickpeas served over Brown Rice

Ingredients:

- ❖ One cup of brown rice
- ❖ One can (15 oz) of rinsed and drained chickpeas

- ❖ One bell pepper
- ❖ 2 Carrots - diced
- ❖ 1 diced Zucchini
- ❖ 1 diced Onion
- ❖ Two diced Garlic cloves
- ❖ One tablespoon minced fresh ginger
- ❖ 1 can (14 oz) milk from coconuts
- ❖ Curry powder - 2 teaspoons
- ❖ One teaspoon of cumin powder
- ❖ One tsp finely ground coriander
- ❖ ½ a teaspoon of turmeric
- ❖ Salt and pepper
- ❖ Two teaspoons vegetable oil
- ❖ **For garnish,** fresh cilantro *is optional*.

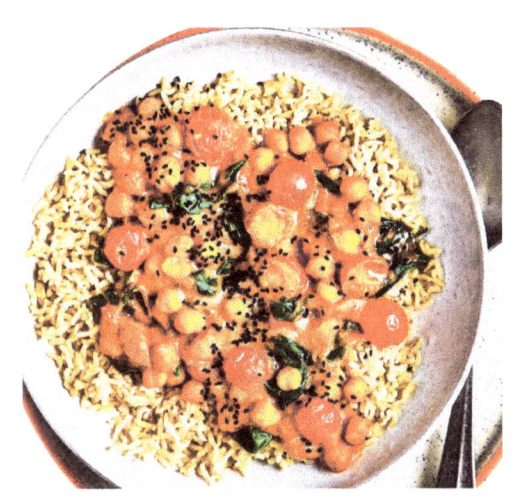

Instruction:

Follow the directions on the box to cook the brown rice, when done - set aside. In a big pan or pot, warm the vegetable oil over medium heat.

Add the chopped onion and simmer for approximately 5 minutes or until transparent.

Add the grated ginger and minced garlic and simmer for an additional minute or until fragrant.
Add curry powder, turmeric, ground coriander, cumin and pepper to taste.
Spices should be cooked for a few minutes to release their aroma. To the pan, add the chopped bell pepper, carrots and zucchini and cook the veggies until they are soft - approximately 5 to 7 minutes.

Add the drained chickpeas and coconut milk. Mix well to combine.

After bringing the mixture to a simmer, cook it for a further 10 to 15 minutes, stirring now and again, until the flavours have blended and the curry has slightly thickened.

If needed, adjust the seasoning by tasting it.

Place the cooked brown rice on top of the veggie curry.
If desired, garnish with fresh cilantro.

Savour your delectable Brown Rice-served Vegetable Curry with Chickpeas.

You are welcome to change the veggies and spices to suit your tastes. This is a very flexible dish; feel free to substitute additional veggies, such as potatoes, spinach or cauliflower.

SNACKS OPTIONS:

Apple slices with Almond Butter

Ingredients:

- ❖ 2 Apples - medium-sized
- ❖ Almond butter
- ❖ **Optional** Toppings *(such chopped nuts, shredded coconut, honey or cinnamon)*

Instruction:

After giving the apples a good cleaning, pat dry with a fresh kitchen towel.

After cored, cut the apples into rounds that are ¼ to ½ inch thick by slicing them horizontally.

The apple peel may be removed *if you'd like*, but keeping it on provides more nutrients and fibre. Top each apple slice with a dollop of almond butter.

Almonds may be blended until smooth to produce your own almond butter or you can use store-bought.

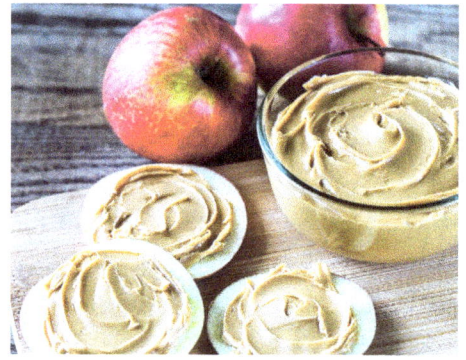

For extra sweetness, you may sprinkle a little honey over the almond butter *if you'd like*.

For added taste and texture, top with chopped nuts, shredded coconut or cinnamon.

Serve the apple slices as a nutritious snack or dessert right away after arranging them on a platter.

Carrot Sticks with Hummus

Ingredients:

- ❖ 2 big carrots
- ❖ 1 can (15 ounces) of rinsed and drained chickpeas
- ❖ Twice as much tahini
- ❖ 2 minced garlic cloves
- ❖ One lemon's juice
- ❖ 2 to 3 teaspoons of extra virgin olive oil
- ❖ Salt to taste.
- ❖ *Add other optional spices*, such Cumin or Paprika - to enhance the flavour.
- ❖ **Garnish optional** fresh parsley or cilantro.

Instructions:

Get the carrot sticks ready:

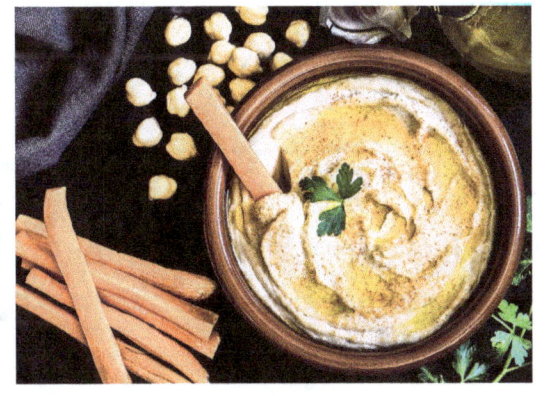

Thoroughly wash the carrots under running water.

After peeling, cut the carrots into 3–4 inch sticks.

Prepare the Hummus:

Put the rinsed and drained chickpeas, tahini, lemon juice, chopped garlic and a dash of salt in a food processor.

Pulse the mixture until it's thoroughly blended and beginning to smooth out.

Olive oil should be added gradually while the food processor is operating, until the hummus has the consistency you want.

Periodically, you may need to scrape down the bowl's sides.

After tasting the hummus, adjust the seasoning by adding extra lemon juice or salt as necessary. For added flavour, you may also add spices like cumin or paprika.

Serve: Move the hummus into a dish for serving. Place the carrot sticks so that they may be dipped around the bowl.

Add some chopped fresh parsley or cilantro and a dab of olive oil to the hummus, *if you'd like.*

Savour your hummus-topped carrot sticks right away. You can change the ingredients to suit your tastes since this recipe is quite adaptable. For added taste and texture, you may also top with extras like pine nuts, roasted red peppers or olives.

Greek Yoghurt with a drizzle of Honey/Maple Syrup

Ingredients:

- ❖ Greek yoghurt *(you may have it plain or flavoured, as you choose)*
- ❖ Honey or Maple syrup

Instruction:

Transfer the necessary quantity of Greek yoghurt into a cup or serving dish.

Drizzle honey over yoghurt with a spoon. The quantity of honey may be changed to suit your own tastes.

If preferred, softly stir the honey into the yoghurt to blend it or leave it as a drizzle over the top.

Savour your Greek yoghurt with honey for a filling and delectable breakfast or snack.

Optional: For added taste and texture, you may also top with extras like granola, almonds or fresh fruit.

Trail Mix with Nuts and Dried Fruit

Ingredients:

- One cup of almonds
- One cup cashews
- One cup of walnuts
- 1 cup of peanuts
- 1 cup of cranberries, dried
- 1 cup of raisins
- 1 cup of chopped dried apricots
- 1 cup of chopped dry mango

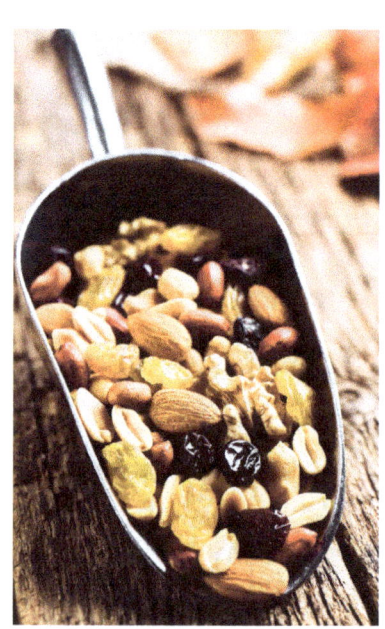

❖ One cup of *optional* Dark chocolate pieces or chips

Instruction:

Set the oven temperature to 350°F (175°C).
Arrange the peanuts, cashews, walnuts and almonds in a single layer on a baking sheet.

For 8 to 10 minutes or until they are aromatic and faintly brown, roast the nuts in the preheated oven.

To avoid burning them, keep a watch on them.

After roasting, take the nuts out of the oven and allow them to cool fully.

The roasted nuts, dried cranberries, raisins, sliced mango, chopped apricots and dark chocolate chunks or chips, *if used,* should all be combined in a big bowl.

Mix everything until well incorporated.

For a maximum of 2 weeks, keep the trail mix at room temperature in an airtight container.

You may alter this recipe by substituting your preferred dried fruits, nuts or seeds. Also, you may change the amounts to suit your tastes.

Cottage Cheese with Pineapple chunks

Ingredients:

- ❖ One cup cottage cheese
- ❖ One cup of fresh pineapple chunks *(if fresh aren't available, you may substitute canned pineapple pieces)*
- ❖ One to two teaspoons of maple syrup or honey *(optional, for sweetness)*
- ❖ A small amount of finely chopped nuts *(optional; adds crunch)*
- ❖ Garnish with fresh mint leaves *(optional).*

Instruction:

Cut the pineapple into tiny bits after peeling and core it if it's fresh.

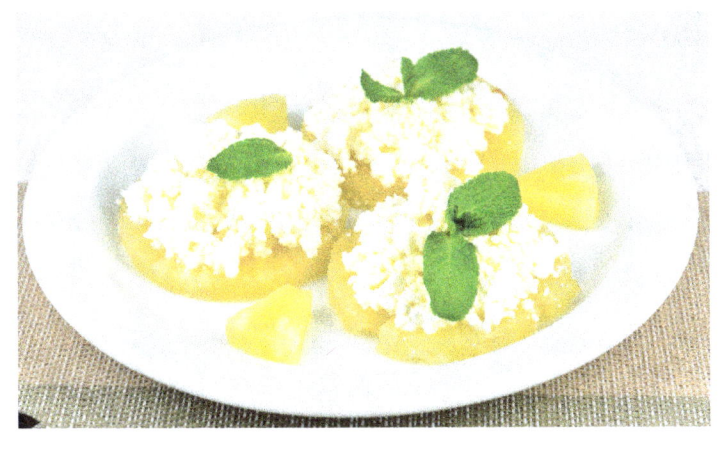

Remove the pineapple pieces from the syrup if using canned pineapple. Place the pineapple pieces and cottage cheese in a mixing dish. You may sweeten the mixture by adding honey or maple syrup, *if you want.*

To suit your taste, start with one tablespoon and work your way up from there.

Once the pineapple pieces are uniformly distributed throughout the cottage cheese, gently mix in the other ingredients.

Add some chopped nuts to the top for flavour and texture *if you'd like.*

Serve the chilled or room temperature cottage cheese and pineapple combination.

If desired, add some fresh mint leaves as a garnish for a cooling effect. Savour it as a dessert, light supper or snack.

You may change the sweetness of this recipe to suit your taste or add other ingredients, such as dried fruit or shredded coconut.

Whole Grain Crackers with Guacamole

Ingredients:

- ❖ Two ripe avocados
- ❖ one juiced lime
- ❖ one-fourth cup finely chopped onions
- ❖ One medium tomato, chopped
- ❖ One tiny jalapeño pepper, chopped finely *(optional for added heat)*
- ❖ 2 minced garlic cloves
- ❖ Salt and pepper.
- ❖ Chop some fresh cilantro *(optional).*

Instruction:

Remove the pits from the avocados, cut them in half, and scoop the flesh into a mixing bowl.

Using a fork, mash the avocado until it's smooth or the consistency you want.

To keep the mashed avocado from browning, add the lime juice and stir well.
Add the minced garlic, tomato, chopped onion and jalapeño *(if using)* and stir.

Add salt and pepper to taste while preparing the guacamole.

Add chopped cilantro for flavour, **if preferred**.

Serve the guacamole right away, accompanied with whole grain crackers for dipping.

Edamame sprinkled with Sea Salt

Ingredients:

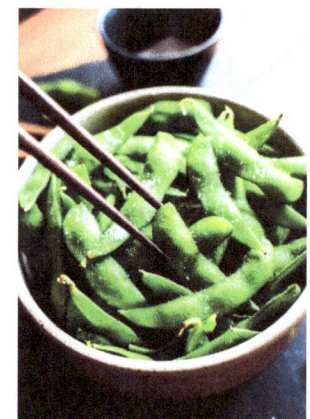

* ❖ One pound or around 450 grams of pod-based Edamame.
* ❖ 1 or 2 teaspoons of sea salt, or to taste
* ❖ Boiling water

Instructions:

If using frozen edamame, thaw it.

Pour water into a big saucepan and heat it until it boils.

When the water is boiling, add the edamame pods and cook for 5 to 7 minutes or until they are soft.

Use a colander to drain the cooked edamame. To remove extra moisture, spread the cooked edamame on paper towels or a clean kitchen towel.

After cooking, move the edamame to a serving basin.

Toss the edamame carefully to ensure that it is uniformly coated after adding the sea salt. Serve as an appetiser or snack.

Avocado slices on Whole Grain Toast

Ingredients:

- ❖ One mature avocado
- ❖ Two pieces of whole grain bread
- ❖ Salt and pepper.
- ❖ *Extra toppings at your discretion:* feta cheese, sliced tomatoes, red pepper flakes or poached eggs

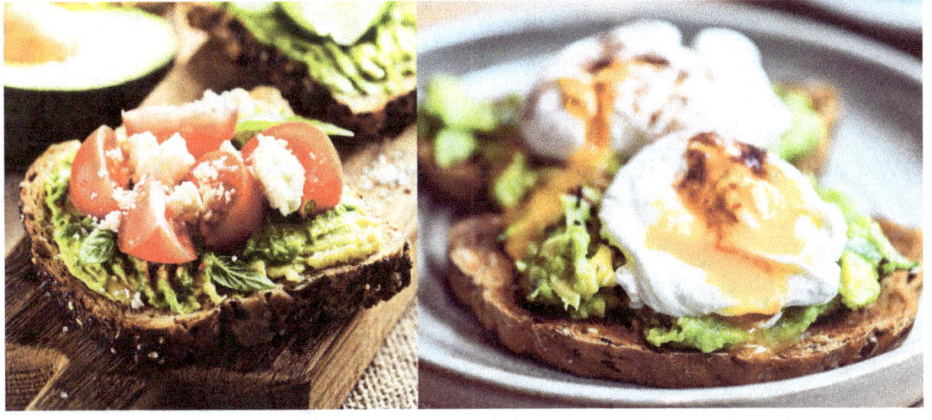

Instruction:

Toasted whole grain bread pieces are the first to take on the ideal crispness.

Cut the avocado in half and remove the pit while the bread is browning. Scoop the avocado flesh into a bowl using a spoon.

Mash the avocado with a fork to the consistency that you like. Depending on your desire, you may either make it smooth or leave it somewhat lumpy.

To taste, add salt and pepper to the mashed avocado and stir well.

When the bread is done, equally distribute the mashed avocado over each piece.

For extra taste and nutrition, you may top the avocado toast with chopped tomatoes, crumbled feta cheese, red pepper flakes or poached eggs, *if you'd like.*

Serve your tasty and nourishing avocado slices on whole grain bread.

Feel free to modify the flavours and toppings to your own taste since this dish is very adaptable.

Cheese and Whole Grain Crackers

Ingredients:

- ❖ 1 cup of flour, whole wheat
- ❖ 1 cup of flour for all purposes
- ❖ One-half tsp baking powder
- ❖ Half a teaspoon of salt
- ❖ 1/4 tsp powdered garlic *(optional)*
- ❖ 1/4 tsp powdered onion *(optional)*
- ❖ 1/4 tsp paprika *(may be added)*
- ❖ 1/4 cup cubed cold unsalted butter
- ❖ One cup of sharp cheddar cheese, shredded
- ❖ 1/4 cup of cold water

Instruction: **Warm up the oven:** Set aside a baking sheet that has been lightly greased or lined with parchment paper and preheat the oven to 375°F (190°C).

Combine the whole wheat flour, all-purpose flour, baking powder, salt and any optional spices *(paprika, onion powder and garlic powder)* in a large mixing bowl.

Add Butter: Mix the flour mixture with the chilled cubed butter. Until the mixture resembles coarse crumbs, cut the butter into the flour with a pastry cutter or your fingertips.

Add Cheese: Using a whisk, stir in the cheddar cheese shreds until they are mixed in completely.

Stirring constantly, gradually pour in the cold water until the dough comes together. The dough may need to be carefully worked into a smooth ball with your hands.

Roll out the dough to a thickness of approximately 1/4 inch on a surface dusted with flour.

Cut the dough into individual crackers of the size and shape you like

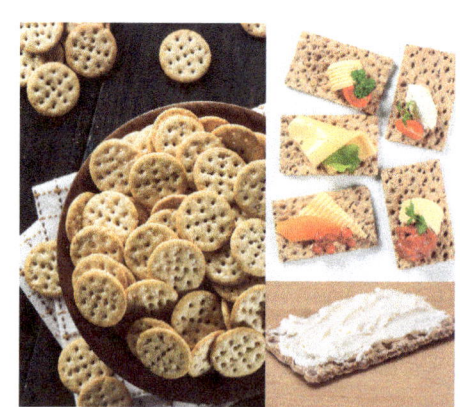

using a knife or cookie cutter.

Spread out the crackers with a little space between them on the baking sheet that has been prepared.

Bake: Bake the crackers for 12 to 15 minutes, or until they are crispy and golden brown, in a preheated oven.

Serve: Let the crackers cool for a few minutes on the baking sheet, then move them to a wire rack to finish cooling. After it cools, serve.

These whole grain and cheese crackers are great as an independent snack or served with your preferred spreads or dips. Any leftovers may be kept for up to a week at room temperature in an airtight container.

Mixed Berries with a dollop of Greek Yoghurt

Ingredients:

- ❖ 1 cup of mixed berries, including blackberries, raspberries, blueberries and strawberries
- ❖ ½ a cup of Greek yoghurt

- ❖ One spoonful of honey, **if desired**
- ❖ Garnish with fresh mint leaves *(optional)*.

Instruction:

After giving the mixed berries a good wash in cold water, blot them dry with paper towels.
Slice the strawberries and remove the stems if you're using them.

Gently stir the Greek yoghurt and honey *(if using)* in a bowl until well blended. Although it's optional, the honey gives the yoghurt a hint of sweetness.

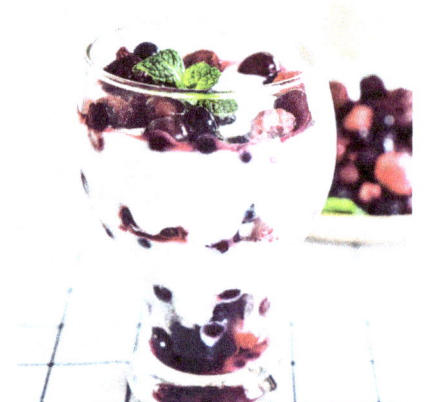

Making a little dollop in the middle of each serving dish or glass, spoon the Greek yoghurt into them.

Layer the mixed berries on top of or around the edges of the yoghurt dollop as you arrange them.

If preferred, garnish with fresh mint leaves for a burst of colour and extra flavour.

Serve right away and enjoy as a wholesome alternative for dessert, brunch or snack.

You may certainly modify this recipe to suit your tastes by changing the amount of yoghurt and berries. If you want more crunch and texture, you may also add additional toppings like granola, almonds or seeds.

SANDWICHES:

Turkey and Cranberry Sandwich on Whole Grain Bread

Ingredients:

- ❖ 4 pieces of whole grain bread
- ❖ 8 pieces Turkey breast - cooked
- ❖ A quarter of a cup of cranberry sauce
- ❖ 4 leaves of lettuce
- ❖ 4 tomato slices and four optional red onion slices
- ❖ Salt and pepper.

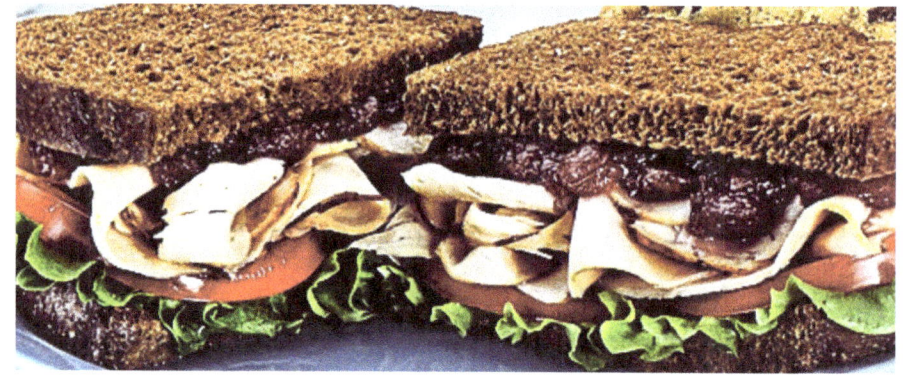

Instruction:

Toast the whole grain bread pieces until they reach the desired crispness.

After toasting, arrange the slices on a spotless surface.

Evenly spread each piece of bread with a spoonful of cranberry sauce.

Top two of the bread pieces with cranberry sauce and two slices of roasted turkey breast.

Add a dash of salt and pepper to taste and season the turkey. Place a tomato slice and a lettuce leaf over the turkey then place a piece of red onion over the tomato *if you'd like*.

To finish the sandwiches, place the remaining bread pieces with cranberry sauce on top. Depending on your choice, cut the sandwiches in half diagonally or straight across.

Your delectable turkey and cranberry sandwiches are ready to be served.

You may add other ingredients, like avocado, cheese or bacon to make this dish your own. Moreover, you may change the amounts of each component to suit your tastes.

Chicken Salad Sandwich with Greek Yoghurt and Grapes on Whole Wheat Bread

Ingredients:
For the Chicken Salad:

- ❖ 2 cups of cooked, chopped or shredded chicken breast
- ❖ Half a cup of plain Greek yoghurt
- ❖ 1/4 cup finely diced red onion
- ❖ 1/4 cup finely chopped celery
- ❖ 1/4 cup of halved, seedless grapes

- ❖ 1/4 cup almonds, slivered *(optional)*
- ❖ One tablespoon of lemon juice
- ❖ Salt and pepper.

For the Sandwich:
- ❖ 4 pieces of whole wheat bread
- ❖ Lettuce stems
- ❖ Tomato slices *(optional)*

Instructions:

Greek yoghurt, diced or shredded chicken breast, red onion, celery, grapes, slivered almonds *(if used)*, and lemon juice should all be combined in a mixing dish. Stir well to coat all ingredients equally.

To taste, add salt and pepper for seasoning.

If preferred, toast the whole wheat bread pieces.

Arrange the lettuce leaves onto a pair of bread pieces.

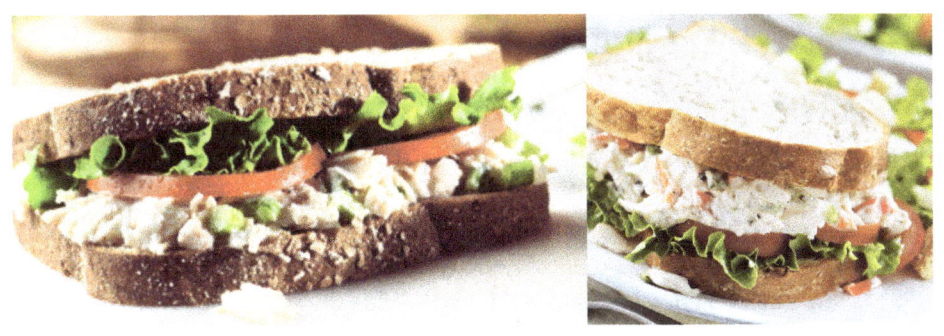

Evenly spoon mixture of chicken salad onto leaves of lettuce.

If you're using tomato slices, arrange them over the chicken salad. To construct sandwiches, place the remaining pieces of bread on top.

If preferred, cut the sandwiches in half diagonally and serve right away.

Veggie Wrap with Hummus, Cucumber, Bell peppers and Spinach in a Whole Wheat Tortilla

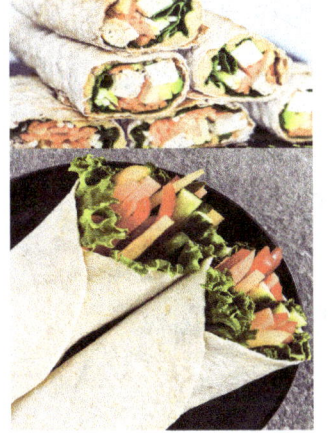

Ingredients:

- ❖ One tortilla made entirely with whole wheat

- ❖ Two tsp of hummus
- ❖ 1/4 of a cucumber, thinly sliced
- ❖ 1/4 of a red bell pepper, cut thinly
- ❖ 1/4 of a yellow bell pepper, cut thinly
- ❖ A handful of fresh spinach leaves
- ❖ Salt and pepper to taste *(if desired)*.

Instruction:

Place the whole wheat tortilla in a flat, tidy heap.

Over the tortilla, equally distribute the hummus, leaving a half-inch border all around.

Arrange the cucumber slices, red, yellow and green bell pepper slices, as well as spinach leaves, on the hummus.

To add more flavour, feel free to season the vegetables with a little salt and pepper.

To wrap the contents, carefully fold the tortilla in half along the sides and roll it securely from the bottom.

Depending on your desire, cut the wrap in half diagonally or leave it intact.

You may either serve it right away or pack it firmly in foil or parchment paper to eat it later.

You can alter it by adding your own vegetables or toppings, such as avocado, shredded carrots or sprouts.

Egg Salad Sandwich on Whole Grain Toast

Ingredients:

- ❖ 6 hard-boiled eggs
- ❖ 1/4 cup of mayonnaise
- ❖ Two teaspoons of finely sliced red onion
- ❖ 1 tablespoon of Dijon mustard
- ❖ 2 teaspoons of celery, finely chopped
- ❖ Salt and pepper.
- ❖ 8 pieces of whole grain bread
- ❖ Leaves from lettuce *(optional)*
- ❖ Tomatoes, cut *(optional)*

Instruction:

The hard-boiled eggs should first be peeled and then cut into tiny pieces. Transfer them into a mixing basin.

To the bowl containing the diced eggs, add the mayonnaise, Dijon mustard, finely sliced red onion and celery.

Once all of the ingredients are fully incorporated, whisk them gently together. To taste, add salt and pepper for seasoning.

Toast the pieces of whole grain bread until they get crispy and golden brown.

When toast is done, top four pieces of toast with a hearty helping of the egg salad mixture.

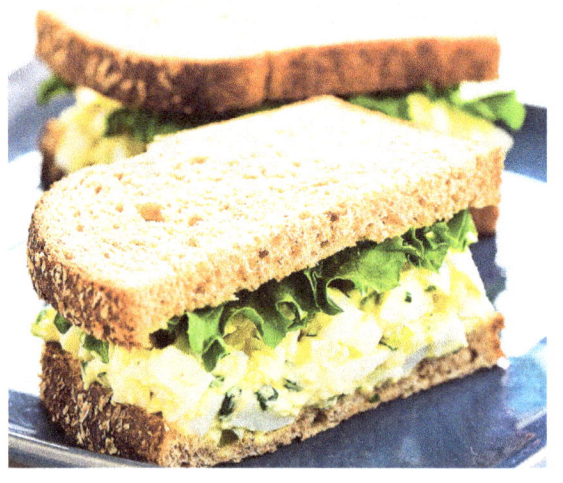

For added taste and texture, you may sprinkle sliced tomatoes and lettuce leaves over the egg salad.

To make sandwiches, place the last four pieces of toast on top.

The egg salad sandwiches may be served right away or stored for later consumption wrapped in foil or parchment paper.

Grilled Cheese Sandwich on Whole Grain Bread with Sliced Tomato

Ingredients:

- ❖ 2 pieces of whole grain bread
- ❖ 2 to 3 pieces of your preferred cheese *(Swiss, mozzarella, cheddar, etc.)*
- ❖ One mature tomato, cut thinly
- ❖ Butter or Margarine
- ❖ *Extra fillings like* fried bacon, avocado pieces, spinach leaves, etc. *are optional*.

Instruction:

In a skillet or frying pan, preheat the heat to medium.

Toast each piece of bread by spreading butter or margarine on one side. Spread butter on one side of the bread piece and place it in the pan.

Cover the whole surface of the bread in the pan with the cheese pieces and place the tomato slices over the cheese.

Spread any extra fillings, *if you'd like,* over the tomato slices.

With the buttered side facing up, place the second piece of bread on top of the contents.

Cook the sandwich for two to three minutes on each side or until the cheese has melted and the bread is golden brown.

Using a spatula, carefully turn the sandwich and cook the other side until golden brown.

Take the sandwich out of the griddle after the cheese has melted and both sides are golden brown.

After allowing it to cool for a minute or two, cut it in half and serve it hot.

Tuna Melt with Avocado and Swiss Cheese on Whole Grain English muffin

Ingredients:

- ❖ One can (5 oz) of drained tuna
- ❖ Mash one ripe avocado.
- ❖ Two split and toasted whole grain English muffins
- ❖ 4 slices of Swiss cheese
- ❖ Salt and pepper.
- ❖ Sliced tomatoes, lettuce and any other toppings you want *are optional.*

Instruction:

Set the grill on high in your oven.

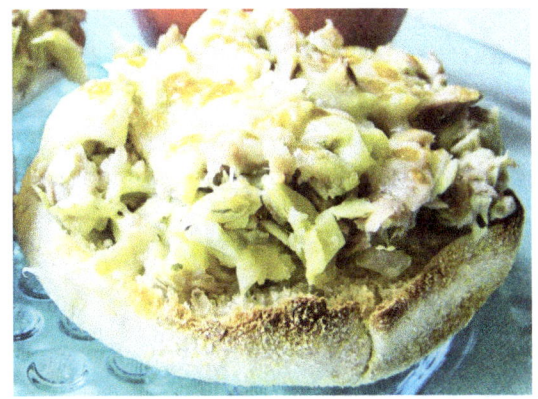

Combine the mashed avocado and the drained tuna in a small bowl. To taste, add salt and pepper for seasoning.

Transfer the English muffin halves to a baking sheet that has been covered with aluminium foil or parchment paper.

Over each half of an English muffin, equally distribute the tuna and avocado mixture and place a
piece of Swiss cheese on top of each muffin half.

Add any other toppings, such as sliced tomatoes or lettuce, *if you'd like*.

When the grill is warmed, place the baking sheet beneath it and broil for 2 to 3 minutes or until the cheese is bubbling and melted.

Take it out of the oven and let it cool down a little before serving.
Warm up some Whole Grain English Muffins with your delectable Tuna Melt with Avocado and Swiss Cheese and enjoy.

Roast Beef and Horseradish Sandwich with Arugula on Whole Grain Ciabatta

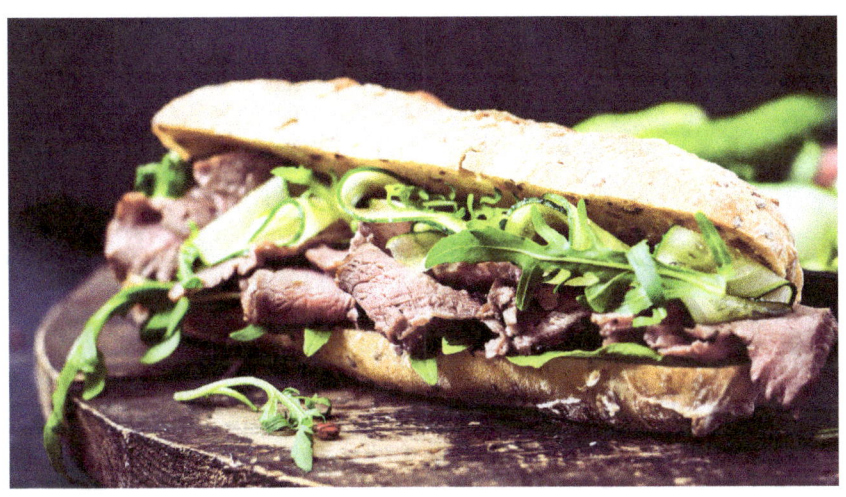

Ingredients:

- ❖ 8 roast beef slices
- ❖ 4 split whole grain ciabatta rolls
- ❖ Half a cup of ready-made horseradish sauce
- ❖ One cup of raw rocket
- ❖ Salt and pepper.

Instruction:

Set the oven temperature to 350°F (175°C).

Spread out the split ciabatta buns on a baking sheet and toast them in the oven for approximately 5 minutes.

Drizzle each roll with a good quantity of horseradish sauce on both halves while the ciabatta toasts.

Arrange the pieces of roast beef equally between the bottom half of the ciabatta buns.

To taste, add salt and pepper to the roast meat.

Sprinkle a handful of fresh rocket leaves over the roast meat.

To make sandwiches, place the upper half of the ciabatta buns on top of the rocket.

Serve your delectable roast beef and horseradish sandwiches on whole grain ciabatta with rocket right away.

Caprese Sandwich with Mozzarella, Tomato, Basil and Balsamic Glaze on Whole Grain Baguette

Ingredients:
- ❖ 1 whole grain baguette

- ❖ 2 ripe tomatoes, thinly sliced
- ❖ 1 huge ball of fresh mozzarella cheese, thinly sliced
- ❖ Fresh basil leaves
- ❖ Balsamic glaze
- ❖ Salt and pepper to taste

Instruction:

Set the oven temperature to 350°F (175°C).

Slice the whole grain bread into appropriate sandwich-sized parts and then slice each piece horizontally to open it up for sandwich creation.

Arrange the bottom half of the baguette slices on a baking sheet and layer the sliced tomatoes on top of the baguette pieces.

Add a layer of thinly sliced fresh mozzarella cheese on top of the tomatoes. Place fresh basil leaves on top of the cheese layer and the drizzle balsamic glaze over the basil leaves.

Sprinkle it with salt and pepper to taste.

Place the top half of the baguette slices on top of the completed sandwiches.

After preheating the oven, place the baking sheet inside and bake for 5 to 10 minutes or until the cheese has melted and the bread has begun to toast slightly.

Once done, remove from the oven and allow to cool for a few minutes before serving.

You can optionally serve with a side salad or some chips for a complete meal.

Hummus and Roasted Vegetable Sandwich on Whole Grain Focaccia

Ingredients:

- ❖ 1 whole grain focaccia bread loaf
- ❖ 1 cup of hummus, homemade or from the store
- ❖ 1 medium aubergine, cut into circles

- ❖ 1 big red pepper cut into slices
- ❖ One medium zucchini cut into lengthwise slices
- ❖ One medium red onion - sliced
- ❖ two teaspoons of olive oil
- ❖ Salt and pepper.
- ❖ 2 cups of mixed salad greens, such spinach or rocket
- ❖ Sliced cucumbers, Tomatoes or any other preferred sandwich ingredients are optional.

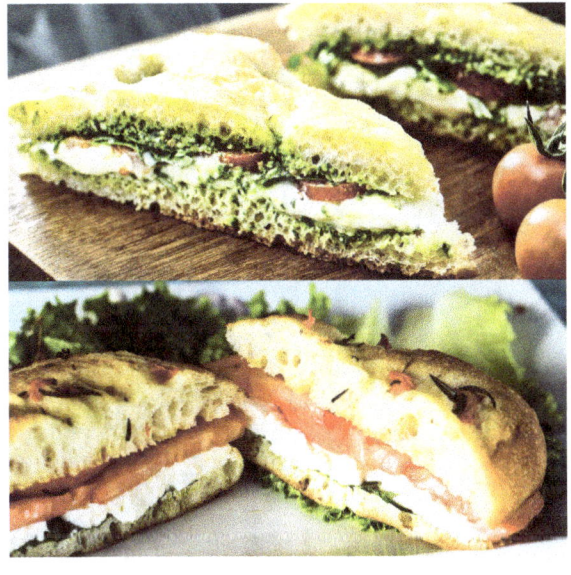

Instructions:

Set oven temperature to 400°F, or 200°C.

Arrange the red onion, zucchini, eggplant and red pepper slices on a baking sheet. Over the veggies, drizzle with olive oil and toss to coat evenly.

To taste, add salt and pepper for seasoning.

When the oven has been preheated, roast the vegetables for 20 to 25 minutes or until they are soft and have begun to caramelise.

After roasting, take the veggies out of the oven and give them a little time to cool.

Make the focaccia: To make a top and bottom piece, slice the whole grain focaccia bread loaf horizontally.

For extra texture, you may optionally bake the focaccia's sliced sides gently in an oven or toaster.

Put the sandwich together:
Drizzle the focaccia bread with a good quantity of hummus on both sliced sides.

Evenly distribute the roasted veggies over the bottom of the focaccia and add mixed salad greens and any other sandwich toppings you like, such cucumber or tomato slices on top of the veggies.

To serve, seal the sandwich by placing the top half of the focaccia bread over the contents.

You may cut the sandwich into separate portions if you'd like.

Smoked Salmon and Cream Cheese with Cucumber slices on Whole Grain Bagel

Ingredients:

- ❖ 1 bagel made with whole grains
- ❖ 2 to 3 ounces of Smoked Salmon
- ❖ 2 to 3 teaspoons of cream cheese
- ❖ 4 or 5 thin slices of Cucumber
- ❖ Dill, fresh *(optional)*
- ❖ Salt and pepper.

Instruction:

Cut the whole grain bagel in half lengthwise,

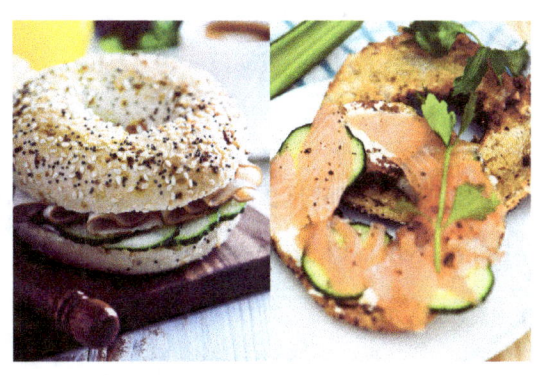

then gently toast it until it becomes somewhat crispy.

Evenly coat both toasted bagel halves with a coating of cream cheese. The quantity of cream cheese may be changed to suit your tastes.

Distribute the smoked salmon over the cream cheese in each of the bagel's two halves.

To make the salmon slices fit perfectly on the bagel, fold them.

Clean the cucumbers, then thinly slice them. Place the cucumber slices over the salmon that has been smoked.

Season the cucumber slices by sprinkling them with a little salt and pepper. *For added flavour,* feel free to add some fresh dill. To assemble, place the remaining bagel half on top to create a sandwich.

Serve: Now that you have your bagel with cream cheese and smoked salmon and cucumber slices, it's time to serve right away.

CONCLUSION

To sum up, this cookbook on Alzheimer's and Dementia health and memory-friendly meals provides a thorough strategy for promoting cognitive health via diet.

Focusing on foods high in antioxidants, good fats and vital minerals makes it a useful tool for people and carers who want to enhance brain health and well-being. The wide variety of dishes, which prioritise components recognised for their cognitive advantages, appeal to a range of tastes and dietary choices - from satisfying soups to nutrient-packed salads and delectable snacks.

People may take proactive measures to preserve brain function and perhaps slow the spread of dementia and Alzheimer's by including these dishes into their regular meal planning.

Bon Appetit!

You can also get the:-
Straight To The Point Alzheimer's Management Guide Made Handy.